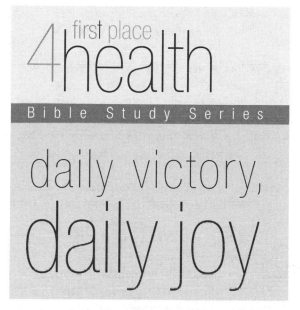

first place
4health

Bible Study Series

daily victory,
daily joy

Published by Gospel Light
Ventura, California, U.S.A.
www.gospellight.com
Printed in the U.S.A.

First Place 4 health Bible study.
p. cm.
#3.— Daily victory, daily joy
ISBN 978-0-8307-4724-5 (trade paper)
1. Bible—Study and teaching. 2. Christian life—Study and teaching.
I. Title: First Place for health Bible study.
BS600.3.F573 2008
242'.5—dc22
2008006856

Rights for publishing this book outside the U.S.A. or in non-English languages
are administered by Gospel Light Worldwide, an international not-for-profit
ministry. For additional information, please visit www.glww.org, email
info@glww.org, or write to Gospel Light Worldwide, 1957 Eastman Avenue,
Ventura, CA 93003, U.S.A.

contents

BIBLE STUDIES

ADDITIONAL MATERIALS

foreword

My introduction to Bible study came when I joined First Place in March 1981. I had been attending church since I was a small child, but the extent of my study of the Bible had been reading my Sunday School quarterly on Saturday night. On Sunday morning, I would listen to my Sunday School teacher as she taught God's Word to me. During the worship service, I would listen to our pastor as he taught God's Word to me. Frankly, digging out the truths of the Bible for myself had never entered my mind.

Perhaps you are right where I was back in 1981. If so, you are in for a blessing you never dreamed possible. As you start studying the truths of the Bible for yourself through the First Place 4 Health Bible studies, you will see God begin to open your understanding of His Word.

Almost every First Place 4 Health member I have talked with about the program says, "The weight loss is wonderful, but the most important thing I have received from my association with First Place 4 Health is learning to study God's Word." The First Place 4 Health Bible studies are designed to be done on a daily basis. As you work through each day's study (which will take 15 to 20 minutes to complete), you will be discovering the deep truths of God's Word. A part of each week's study will also include a Bible memory verse for the week.

There are many in-depth Bible studies on the market. The First Place 4 Health Bible studies are not designed for the purpose of in-depth study, but are designed to be used in conjunction with the rest of the program to bring balance into your life. Our desire is for each member to begin having a personal quiet time with God each day. This time alone with God should include a time of prayer, Bible reading and Bible study. Having a quiet time is a daily discipline that will bring the rich rewards of balance, which is something we all need.

God bless you as you begin this exciting journey toward a balanced life. God will richly bless your efforts to give Him first place in your life. Remember Matthew 6:33: "But seek first his kingdom and his righteousness, and all these things will be given to you as well."

Carole Lewis
First Place 4 Health National Director

introduction

First Place 4 Health is a Christ-centered health program that emphasizes balance in the physical, mental, emotional and spiritual areas of life. The First Place 4 Health program is meant to be a daily process. As we learn to keep Christ first in our lives, we will find that He is the One who satisfies our hunger and our every need.

This Bible study is designed to be used in conjunction with the First Place 4 Health program but can be beneficial for anyone interested in obtaining a balanced lifestyle. The Bible study has been created in a five-day format, with the last two days reserved for reflection on the material studied. Keep in mind that the ultimate goal of studying the Bible is not only for knowledge but also for application and a changed life. Don't feel anxious if you can't seem to find the *correct* answer. Many times, the Word will speak differently to different people, depending on where they are in their walk with God and the season of life they are experiencing. Be prepared to discuss with your fellow First Place 4 Health members what you learned that week through your study.

There are some additional components included with this study that will be helpful as you pursue the goal of giving Christ first place in every area of your life:

- **Group Prayer Request Form:** This form is at the end of each week's study. You can use this to record any special requests that might be given in class.

- **Leader Discussion Guide:** This discussion guide is provided to help the First Place 4 Health leader guide a group through this Bible study. It includes ideas for facilitating a First Place 4 Health class discussion for each week of the Bible study.

- **Two Weeks of Menu Plans with Recipes:** There are 14 days of meals, and all are interchangeable. Each day totals 1,400 to 1,500 calories and includes snacks. Instructions are given for those who need more calories. An accompanying grocery list includes items that will be needed for each week of meals.

- **First Place 4 Health Member Survey:** Fill this out and bring it to your first meeting. This information will help your leader know your interests and talents.

- **Personal Weight and Measurement Record:** Use this form to keep a record of your weight loss. Record any loss or gain on the chart after the weigh-in at each week's meeting.

- **Weekly Prayer Partner Forms:** Fill out this form before class and place it into a basket during the class meeting. After class, you will draw out a prayer request form, and this will be your prayer partner for the week. Try to call or email the person sometime before the next class meeting to encourage that person.

- **Live It Trackers:** Your Live It Tracker is to be completed at home and turned in to your leader at your weekly First Place 4 Health meeting. The Tracker is designed to help you practice mindfulness and stay accountable with regard to your eating and exercise habits. Step-by-step instructions for how to use the Live It Tracker are provided in the *Member's Guide*.

- **Let's Count Our Miles!** A worthy goal we encourage is for you to complete 100 miles of exercise during your 12 weeks in First Place 4 Health. There are many activities listed on pages 255-256 that count toward your goal of 100 miles. When you complete a mile of activity, mark off the box listed on the Hundred Mile Club chart located on the inside of the back cover.

- **Scripture Memory Cards:** These cards have been designed so that you can use them while exercising. It is suggested that you punch a hole in the upper left corner and place the cards on a ring. You may want to take the cards in the car or to work so that you can practice each week's Scripture memory verse throughout the day.

- **Scripture Memory CD:** All 10 Scripture memory verses have been put to music at an exercise tempo in the CD at the back of this study. Use this CD when exercising or even when you are just driving in your car. The words of Scripture are often easier to memorize when accompanied by music.

Use each of these important tools found in this study to live a balanced and healthy life.

welcome to
Daily Victory, Daily Joy

At your first group meeting for this session of First Place 4 Health, you will meet your fellow members, get an overview of your materials and find out what you can expect at weekly meetings. The majority of your class time will be spent learning about the four-sided person concept, the Live It Food Plan, and how change begins from the inside out. You will also have a chance to ask any questions about how to get the most out of First Place 4 Health. If possible, complete the Member Survey on page 205 before your first group meeting. The information you give will help your leader tailor the next 12 weeks to the needs of the whole group.

Each weekly meeting begins with a weigh-in for members. This will allow you to track your progress over the 12-week session. Your Week One weigh-in/measurement will establish a baseline of comparison so that you can set healthy goals for this session. If you are apprehensive about weighing in every week, talk with your group leader about your concerns. He or she will have some options for you to consider that will make the weigh-in activity encouraging rather than stressful.

The day after your first meeting, begin Week Two of this Bible study. This session, you and your group will explore how to set realistic goals for yourself and how to realize the daily joy that comes when you choose to put Christ first in all things in your life. Instead of falling prey to discouragement and doubt and allowing the enemy—who "prowls around like a roaring lion looking for someone to devour" (1 Peter 5:8)—to sabotage your efforts, you can experience victory every day when you and your fellow First Place 4 Health members allow God's Word to show you the way. As you open yourself to the truth of Scripture and share your hopes and struggles with the members of your group during the next 12 weeks, you'll find yourself becoming the healthy child of God that you are designed to be!

not beyond
our reach

SCRIPTURE MEMORY VERSE
*Now what I am commanding you today is not
too difficult for you or beyond your reach.*
DEUTERONOMY 30:11

When we first begin the First Place 4 Health program, it is necessary for us to set goals. These goals allow us to begin with the end in mind, chart our pre-scribed course and take the daily steps that will lead us to our desired destina-tion. However, as necessary as goals are to our success in First Place 4 Health, we need to be careful to not become so focused on the end result that we miss the joy that can be ours today and miss the daily victories found in the process of keeping Christ first in all things.

When we allow ourselves to become obsessed with the destination, it is easy for us to erroneously imagine that on a certain day and at a certain time, we will finally arrive at our desired destination. Day after day, we keep telling ourselves that when that long-awaited moment finally arrives, all our wonderful dreams will immediately come true and the pieces of our lives will suddenly fit together like a completed jigsaw puzzle. We fret and worry and hurry through our days— to get nowhere but to a tomorrow that never comes, because somewhere in the process it becomes today. We spend our lives waiting for the magic moment when our life will really begin—and in our haste, we miss the joy that can be ours in the present moment.

Sooner or later, we will come to realize that there is no final destination un-til we reach the end of our time here on earth. Each goal realized will merely lead to another and then another, and life will take place in the process. Yes, there will be milestones to celebrate, those special days that mark the passage from one leg of the journey to the next. The end will come soon enough, but through it all, the true joy of life is found in the wonder of today.

For many of us in First Place 4 Health, life has been a continuing saga of waiting for the magic moment when we will suddenly see the right number on the scales and our lives can finally begin. *When I lose 50 pounds,* we tell ourselves, *then I'll go back to school. When I can wear a size 10 again, I'll visit my friends who knew me way back when. When my body is smaller, I'll pursue the career I've always dreamed of.* But when we put life on hold, we rob ourselves of daily victory and daily joy.

First Place 4 Health is not about putting life on hold until we reach our physical, mental, emotional and spiritual goals. It is about living in joyful obedience today, trusting that the miracle-in-the-making will unfold as we take the next right step in the right direction. Daily victory and daily joy can be ours when we keep Christ first in all things.

ENCOUNTERING OBSTACLES

Day 1

Lord, as I begin this leg of my journey, I pray You will be with me and help me to overcome the obstacles that stand between me and Your plan for my life. Amen.

When we begin this lifelong journey toward health and wholeness, it is easy for us to become overwhelmed when we think about the future. Not only do we begin to envision that wonderful day when we will reach our goal, we also begin to see the roadblocks and hazards that stand in our path. Soon, we find ourselves fretting about tomorrow rather than enjoying the simple pleasures that are ours today. In Luke 9:51, we read of a transition point in Jesus' earthly ministry that can help us understand the importance of taking the next right step in the right direction and leaving the future in God's hands. Jesus had been ministering in the region around Galilee since the beginning of His ministry. Now, our Savior was about to embark on the final leg of His journey.

Jesus did not just start out for Jerusalem. What word does Luke use to describe how Jesus set out toward His destination?

Jesus _____ set out for Jerusalem.

How can you apply this word to the personal journey toward health and wholeness that you are making in the First Place 4 Health program?

_____

_____

_____

No sooner does Luke tell us that Jesus has resolutely set out for Jerusalem than we learn about an obstacle. Read Luke 9:52-55 and describe what happened.

_____

_____

_____

How might you encounter resistance from others now that you have resolutely set out on the journey toward your wellness goals?

_____

_____

_____

What can you learn from the way Jesus faced the resistance He encountered on His journey to your First Place 4 Health journey?

_____

_____

_____

What would have happened if Jesus had allowed the resistance He encountered to keep Him from making His journey?

_____

_____

_____

What will happen if you allow the resistance of others to keep you from making your personal journey to health, wholeness and a balanced lifestyle that honors God?

_____

_____

_____

Thank You, Loving Lord, for giving me the resolve I will need to face the challenges and obstacles that You know lie ahead of me as I journey toward my First Place 4 Health goals. Amen.

CONSIDER THE COST

Sovereign Lord, help me to honor my pledge to follow You rather than
being numbered among the excuse makers that talk a better game than
they are willing to play. Amen.

In yesterday's lesson, we learned that Jesus *resolutely* set out for Jerusalem. Yet the journey took many months, and as He traveled along the dusty roads between Galilee and Jerusalem, Jesus met, and interacted with, many people. After the Samaritans refused to welcome Him, we are told that He went on to another village. In this village, Jesus encountered another type of resistance.

Turn in your Bible to Luke 9:57-62. What does verse 57 tell us happened as Jesus was walking along the road?

_____

_____

_____

How did Jesus reply to the eager fellow? Why did He answer as He did?

_____

_____

_____

Think of a time when you enthusiastically began a diet and exercise program but weren't given all the details about the obstacles you would encounter along the way. Describe this experience and how you felt when you discovered important information had been withheld—information that might have changed your mind about following the program had you known the truth from the very beginning.

_____

_____

_____

_____

Luke 9:59 tells us about another person Jesus encountered along the road. What did Jesus say to this man, and how did the man reply?

_____

_____

_____

_____

It is easy to misinterpret Jesus' reply and believe He was telling this man not to participate in the burial of his father. However, if we closely examine the man's words, we see that they are really just a thinly veiled excuse. Under the Jewish custom of the day, the deceased were buried before sunset on the day they died. Had the man's father just died, he would not have been traveling along the road where he met Jesus. He would have been busy burying his father! What this man was really asking was for Jesus to allow him to put off following Him until after his father—who may not have even been old or even sick—had died!

How have you put off your physical, mental, emotional and spiritual goals until sometime in the future, when you felt it would be more convenient?

_____

_____

_____

_____

If Jesus heard you offering that excuse, what would He say to you? How would that be like Him telling the man to let the dead bury the dead?

_____

_____

_____

What was this man to do rather than sitting around waiting for his father to die (see Luke 9:60)?

_____

_____

_____

How are you being asked to go and proclaim the kingdom of God through your participation in the First Place 4 Health program?

_____

_____

_____

What excuse are you offering rather than doing what Jesus has asked you to do?

_____

_____

_____

O Gracious God, forgive me for those times I offer You feeble excuses rather than simply following Your instructions to follow You. Amen.

FAMILY OBLIGATIONS

Day 3

Lord, You are not fooled by my excuses. Help me to always see Your requests of me as loving, kind and compassionate rather than burdensome and difficult. Amen.

Yesterday, we looked at two people Jesus encountered as He began His trip from Galilee to Jerusalem. Today we are going to look at a third man—and a different type of resistance.

Turn back in your Bible to Luke 9:61. What does this man say to Jesus?

_____

_____

_____

_____

What was Jesus' reply to this man's words (see Luke 9:62)?

_____

_____

_____

_____

Have you made a commitment to follow a weight-loss program at some time in the past but then allowed family ties and obligations to sabotage your goals?

_____

_____

_____

_____

Two other disciples heard Jesus call them to follow Him. In Mark 1:19-20, who were the disciples Jesus called? What was their response when Jesus asked them to follow Him?

_____

_____

_____

_____

Who did these two men leave behind when Jesus called them?

_____

_____

_____

_____

How is this different from the request of the man in Luke 9:62?

_____

_____

_____

Notice that these two men were working with their father when Jesus called them, while the man in Luke 9:62 was traveling down the road away from his family. How does this make their response even more significant?

_____

_____

_____

_____

What family obligations do you need to let go of in order to follow the First Place 4 Health program? (As you answer this question, remember that the Lord would never ask you to abandon a God-given family responsibility to follow Him. The "obligations" you need to identify are things such as keeping cookies in the cabinet for your children and grandchildren or cooking high-fat meals that no one in your family benefits from eating. These are examples of the types of obligations you will have to give up in order to follow Jesus' command that you care for your body.)

_____

_____

_____

_____

How can your participation in First Place 4 Health benefit all the members of your family? (Think of both their own health and the benefit of having a healthier you in their lives as you answer this question.)

_____

_____

_____

_____

Luke 9:62 gives us an interesting bit of information. What does Jesus say this man had done before he asked to go back and say goodbye to his family?

_____

_____

_____

How have you "put your hand to the plow" when following a weight-loss program in the past and then decided it was too difficult and looked for a way out? What was that way out, and where did it lead you?

_____

_____

_____

_____

What have you learned about the cost of following Jesus as you have read this week's lesson? How will that information have an impact on your First Place 4 Health commitment?

_____

_____

_____

_____

_____

Merciful and compassionate Father, You are not fooled by my excuses. You always ask me to consider the cost before I put my hand to the plow, not enthusiastically begin and then look for a way out. Amen.

Day
4

NO TURNING BACK

Forgive me, gracious God, for the times I make a commitment to You and then turn back when the road gets difficult and I lose sight of the vision that You have put before me. Amen.

In yesterday's lesson, we looked at an excuse-maker who "put his hand to the plow" and then looked back. Hebrews 11 could best be described as the roll call of the faithful saints who have gone before us.

Turn to Hebrews 11:15. What truth do you find in these words?

_____

_____

_____

_____

How was the fellow from yesterday's lesson thinking about the "country he had left" and looking for an opportunity to return?

_____

_____

_____

_____

Since joining First Place 4 Health, have you thought about other diet and exercise programs that you have tried in the past—perhaps programs that produced faster weight loss results? How were you tempted to find an opportunity to return to that program instead of staying in First Place 4 Health?

_____

_____

_____

_____

What convinced you to stay in the First Place 4 Health program? Or are you still looking for a way out of your First Place 4 Health commitment?

_____

_____

_____

What were the people in Hebrews 11:16 longing for?

_____

_____

_____

What was the "better country" you were longing for when you enrolled in the First Place 4 Health program?

_____

_____

_____

Hebrews 11:16 also gives us an important piece of information about how God reacts to those who are not ashamed to follow Him, even when they face opposition. What does Hebrews 11:16 tell us?

_____

_____

_____

_____

Hebrews 11:13 tells us that the faithful followers of God live as though they are aliens and strangers on this earth. How does your participation in First Place 4 Health alienate you from those who continue to live a life characterized by out of control eating and not caring for themselves?

_____

_____

_____

Although you may be tempted from within and from without, there is daily victory and daily joy for those who keep Christ first in all things. Describe one joy you have experienced today as a result of participation in First Place 4 Health. You might want to incorporate the sentiment expressed in Hebrews 11:16 about God's reaction to those who are faithful as you answer this question.

_____

_____

_____

_____

O Sovereign Lord, how thankful I am that You are not ashamed to be called my God and that I can always be confident that You are on this journey with me, even as You prepare a better place for me. Amen.

Day 5 — NOT TOO DIFFICULT

O Lord God, thank You for Your great and precious promise that assures me that what You are asking of me is not too difficult or beyond my reach. Amen.

This week, we have looked at some of the obstacles that can stand between us and faithful obedience to Jesus' command that we follow Him. What have you learned from these lessons?

_____

_____

_____

_____

How will this knowledge help you succeed in your First Place 4 Health efforts?

_____

_____

_____

As you contemplate the cost of discipleship, look at the assurance given in this week's Scripture Memory Verse. Write the memory verse below, and then underline that assurance that is provided.

_____

_____

_____

How is the word "too" key to understanding the truth of Deuteronomy 30:11?

_____

_____

_____

As beneficial as it is to memorize Scripture, it is also important to consider the memory verses in the context in which they are written. How does Deuteronomy 30:12-14 help you understand the meaning of this week's memory verse?

_____

_____

_____

Where is the word according to verse 14?

_____

_____

_____

How do you think the word of God gets into the mouth and heart of God's faithful people?

_____

_____

_____

Deuteronomy 30:15-16 gives us further information about why God has given us His word. According to those verses, what has God set before us in giving us His commandments, decrees and laws?

_____

_____

_____

What is promised for those who love the Lord their God, walk in His ways and keep His commandments, decrees and laws (see Deuteronomy 30:16)?

_____

_____

_____

How has God set life and prosperity before you? How is participation in First Place 4 Health part of loving the Lord your God, walking in His ways and keeping His commandments?

_____

_____

_____

Now look at Deuteronomy 30:19. What has God put before you?

_____

_____

_____

Which do you choose today: life or death, blessing or curses? How could your faithful participation in First Place 4 Health be part of that choice?

_____

_____

_____

O Lord God, this day You have put life and death before me. Help me to choose life by faithfully following Your commands as I walk in Your ways and love You with all my heart, mind, spirit and strength. Amen.

REFLECTION AND APPLICATION

Lord, You continue to set before me life and death. Today I choose to enjoy the good things You have given me to make the journey as exciting as the results. Amen.

In the introduction to this week's lesson, we looked at some of the things we often put on hold until we reach our wellness goals: "When I lose 50 pounds, then I'll go back to school," "When I can wear a size 10 again I'll visit my friends who knew me way back when," "When my body is smaller, I'll pursue the career I've always dreamed of." And although these words probably have generic application to all our lives, each one of us has specific dreams that we have put on hold until we reach our ideal body weight.

What are the things you are putting off until that magical day when you suddenly have the body you've always dreamed of? In the space below, complete all six of the "when I lose weight, then I will" statements.

1. When I lose weight, then I will _____

2. When I lose weight, then I will _____

3. When I lose weight, then I will _____

4. When I lose weight, then I will _____

5. When I lose weight, then I will _____

6. When I lose weight, then I will _____

Now go back and analyze the list you have just made. What is stopping you from doing these things, even as you work to achieve your wellness goals?

_____

_____

_____

_____

_____

_____

O God, forgive me for putting off until tomorrow the things You have given me to enjoy today. Amen.

Day
7

REFLECTION AND APPLICATION

O Lord God, all too often I make excuses rather than finding solutions that allow me to walk in Your ways and obey Your commands. Forgive me for finding ways of turning back rather than remaining faithful to You. Amen.

In our Day Three study, we looked at some "family obligations" that often keep us from being faithful to our commitment to our physical, mental, spiritual and emotional health. Go back to that day's lesson and review the obligations you listed. Now expand that list so that you have five family obligations that have the potential to hinder your First Place 4 Health efforts. As you look at the list, find five creative solutions to those obligations that will allow you to care for your family but still keep to your wellness goals.

Family Obligation that Threatens My First Place 4 Health Program	Creative Solution

O great and awesome God, thank You for giving me creative solutions to the problems that threaten my success in the First Place 4 Health program. Amen.

Group Prayer Requests

4 first place
health

Today's Date: _____

Name	Request

Results

_____
_____
_____
_____
_____
_____
_____

words for the wise traveler

When many of us first begin our First Place 4 Health journey, we are full of energy and enthusiasm. Visions of finally achieving our fitness goals fill our hearts and minds with hope. In our zeal, we vow that this time will be different—this time we won't allow people, places and things to interfere with our plans and dreams. As we have seen, all too often those plans are derailed.

Pause for a moment and think about your hopes and dreams for this session of First Place 4 Health. Where do you envision yourself 10 weeks from now—not just physically, but also in the other aspects of your being? Be specific about your goals and expectations in the following areas:

Physically _____

_____

_____

Mentally _____

_____

_____

Emotionally _____

_____

_____

Spiritually _____

_____

_____

Maybe you are skeptical even as you write out these goals. Perhaps you have made vows regarding your wellness goals before but encountered obstacles you had not planned for. Perhaps you had not anticipated just how powerful the hold food had over you—or the power of the negative voices that told you that you couldn't have victory over this area of your life. All too soon, your grand hopes and dreams came crashing down around you as the daily challenges of life stood between you and the vows you made when your motivation was high and your enthusiasm was fresh and new.

What was the last vow you made regarding your physical, mental, emotional and spiritual health, and what was the end result?

_____

_____

_____

If your life has been a series of broken vows when it comes to achieving your wellness goals, take heart! You can emerge victorious from the inner battle that has kept you in doubt, defeat and despair. God has a plan for you, and that plan is good. There can be daily victory and daily joy. Jesus has overcome the world, and in His might and power, you can overcome as well.

WISE WORDS ON TAKING VOWS

Day 1

O Lord, forgive me for the times I have made a vow to You and then not fulfilled it. Forgive me for letting other things stand between me and doing Your will. Amen.

In Matthew 5:37, Jesus cautioned, "Simply let your 'Yes' be 'Yes' and your 'No' be 'No,' for anything beyond this comes from the evil one." How do Jesus' words affirm the truth of this week's memory verse?

_____

_____

_____

Now look at Matthew 5:33. How is the saying Jesus quotes in this verse similar to our memory verse for this week?

_____

_____

_____

_____

In Matthew 5:34-35, Jesus tells us that there is a better way. Paraphrase what Jesus is saying in those verses in your own words.

_____

_____

_____

_____

Why do you think Jesus emphasizes the fact that we can't even make one hair on our head white or black?

_____

_____

_____

_____

How does this saying correspond to Jesus' words in Matthew 6:25-27?

_____

_____

_____

_____

If we are not to swear or take oaths or worry about what we will eat or drink, what are we to do (see Matthew 6:33)?

_____

_____

_____

_____

How is this different from making a vow?

_____

_____

_____

_____

James gives us more advice about taking vows. He calls making vows bragging and boasting about tomorrow. Turn in your Bible to James 4:13-17 and read James's words. How does this passage correspond with Matthew 5:34-35 and Matthew 6:25-27?

_____

_____

_____

_____

Considering what Jesus and James have to say about the danger of making oaths or taking vows, why do you think Jesus tells us to simply let our yes be yes and our no be no?

_____

_____

_____

_____

Jesus tells us that anything beyond this comes from the evil one—the one who is trying to lead us astray. What have you learned about making vows during today's lesson that affirm Jesus' words on taking oaths?

_____

_____

_____

_____

O Lord God, You are the one who holds my future and sees my tomorrows. Thank You for allowing me to leave the details to You so that I can simply say yes to Your request that I follow You. Amen.

Day 2

BOASTING OR FOLLOWING

Sovereign Lord, forgive me for those times I fail to say no to the things of the world that interfere with my saying yes to You. Amen.

Yesterday, we looked at the importance of letting our yes be yes and our no be no. Summarize what you learned about taking vows from yesterday's lesson:

_____

_____

_____

How is saying yes to Jesus' call to follow Him different from making a vow?

_____

_____

_____

During last week's study, we read about two fishermen who responded to Jesus' simple call to come and follow Him. What did James and John do when Jesus called them?

_____

_____

_____

Mark 1:16-18 tells us that Jesus also called to two other men that day. What are the names of these men, and what were their relationship and their occupation?

_____

_____

_____

Mark 1:18 tells us what these two men did in response to Jesus' words. Write out verse 18 and then underline the first two words of the sentence.

_____

_____

_____

How are these words different from boasting about something that will be done in the future?

_____

_____

_____

_____

How would you describe your First Place 4 Health participation? When you heard Jesus calling you to pursue a healthier lifestyle, did you clear your calendar so that you could do as Jesus asked? Or are you still just talking about what you will do? Explain your answer.

_____

_____

_____

_____

_____

_____

Recall the advice James gave us in yesterday's lesson. James ends his counsel with the words, "Anyone, then, who knows the good he ought to do and doesn't do it, sins" (James 4:17). What do you know that you should be doing when it comes to your wellness that you are not doing? Why aren't you taking action?

_____

_____

_____

_____

How is making a vow different from taking action? How does this explain why Jesus said anything more than simply saying yes or no is from the evil one?

_____

_____

_____

_____

What have you given up so that you can wholeheartedly commit yourself to physical, mental, emotional and spiritual fitness through participation in First Place 4 Health?

_____

_____

_____

What are the things you must leave behind in order to achieve success about letting your yes be yes and your no be no?

_____

_____

_____

What do you need to say no to in order to say yes to Jesus' call that you care for yourself as a reflection of His love for you?

_____

_____

_____

_____

_____

O Lord, how foolish I am when I make vows instead of simply saying yes to the things You are asking of me. Please forgive me for substituting boastful words for consistent action. Amen.

Day 3 — HEEDING JESUS' WARNING

Loving Lord, thank You for showing me the way to lead a life pleasing to You. Help me to learn the lesson You have for me today in this study. Amen.

Three years after Peter answered Jesus' call to follow Him and become a fisher of men, Peter was faced with another situation in which he had to make a choice. Jesus and the disciples had just shared the Passover meal together, and Jesus was trying to prepare the disciples for what would happen during the next 24 hours. At the conclusion of this meal, Jesus gave Peter a warning.

Turn to Luke 22:31-32. Read what Jesus is saying to Peter in these verses, and then summarize them in your own words.

_____

_____

_____

Rather than listening to Jesus' words of warning, Peter did something else. Read Luke 22:33. What did Peter do instead?

_____

_____

_____

How is the Lord warning you about the dangers you will encounter on the road to health and wholeness?

_____

_____

_____

_____

Are you listening to Jesus' words of warning, or are you "boasting" about what you can do in your own might and power? Explain your answer.

_____

_____

_____

_____

What specific word of warning have you heard the Lord speaking to you so far during this study? We have looked at many pitfalls, so pick the one that you feel the Holy Spirit has impressed most deeply on your heart.

_____

_____

_____

_____

How did you respond to that warning? Did you heed Jesus' words and take the necessary steps to protect yourself, or have you turned a deaf ear and decided to do things "your way"?

_____

_____

_____

Jesus did not argue with Peter when Peter chose not to listen to His words. How did He respond to Peter's boast (see Luke 22:34)?

_____

_____

_____

A few short hours after Peter's boast, his words were put to the test—and Jesus' prediction came to pass. Turn to Luke 22:54-62. This is a familiar story to most of us, so read it with new eyes to see where taking vows can lead. What happened to Peter?

_____

_____

_____

How have the vows you made in the past about accomplishing your health and weight-loss goals had similar results? Tell about a recent time when your "boasting" lead to disaster in your life.

_____

_____

_____

Jesus told Peter that Satan had asked to sift him like wheat. What had Jesus done in response to Satan's request?

_____

_____

_____

How can the awareness that Jesus is praying for you be a source of strength and encouragement as you continue your journey to health, balance and a lifestyle that is pleasing to God?

_____

_____

_____

_____

_____

Gracious Lord, thank You for praying for me even though You can see where my self-sufficiency will lead me. Thank You for restoring me when I fail. Amen.

A BOAST THAT LEADS TO DISASTER

Day
4

Gracious God, it is so easy for me to cave in to the pressure of others rather than seeking to always do what is pleasing to You. Please forgive me. Amen.

John the Baptist was the forerunner sent to announce the coming of the Messiah. When John was asked who he was, he described himself as "the voice of one calling in the desert, 'Make straight the way for the Lord'" (John 1:23).

How is God using the First Place 4 Health program to call you back to paths that are pleasing to the Lord?

_____

_____

_____

_____

John the Baptist boldly confronted those who were living contrary to God's word and will. As a result, he was thrown into prison. Read the story of John's arrest and imprisonment in Matthew 14:3-5. Why was Herod afraid to kill John?

_____

_____

_____

_____

Read Matthew 14:6-7. What did Herod vow to do when the daughter of Herodias pleased him with her dancing?

_____

_____

_____

What was the thing her mother prompted her to ask for?

_____

_____

_____

Matthew 14:9 tells us that King Herod was _____ when he heard the request. Yet he did as the girl asked. Why did Herod grant the request?

_____

_____

_____

Herod was what we would today call a "people-pleaser." At first, he refused to kill John because he feared the people, then later he beheaded John because he feared the reaction of his birthday dinner guests. How has being a people-pleaser caused you to make vows that you could not keep or that were harmful to you when you kept them?

_____

_____

_____

How can being a people-pleaser create problems in your journey toward health and wholeness?

_____

_____

_____

Read Matthew 6:33, the foundational verse of the First Place 4 Health program, if you don't know it from memory. How can the instructions given in this verse keep us from the people-pleasing we do that keeps us from pleasing God?

_____

_____

_____

_____

O Lord God, when I seek first Your kingdom and Your righteousness, I am not concerned with the actions and reactions of others. Thank You for showing me the pathway that leads to life. Amen.

MANY WORDS ARE MEANINGLESS

Day
5

Lord, all too often I fail to put my words into meaningful action. Help me to follow through on my commitments and keep You at the center of my life. Amen.

Our Week Three memory verse comes from the book of Ecclesiastes. In this book, the "Teacher" looks at wisdom, pleasure, work, power, riches, religion and a number of other things that have some value. But, as he ultimately discovers, these things are only useful in their proper time and place and only have lasting value if God is at the center of a person's life.

How does this correspond with what you read in Matthew 6:33 during yesterday's study?

_____

_____

_____

Write this week's memory verse below. (By now, you should be able to write it from memory!)

_____

_____

_____

_____

In order to correctly understand the meaning of this verse, we must look at it in the context in which it appears in the Bible. So turn to Ecclesiastes 5 and read verses 4-7. What new information can you glean from these verses that gives deeper meaning to the words contained in Ecclesiastes 5:5?

_____

_____

_____

During our Week Two study, we heard Jesus talk about those who had put their hand to the plow and then looked back (see Luke 9:62). How does Ecclesiastes 5:6 address the same problem?

_____

_____

_____

When have you made a vow regarding a specific diet or exercise plan that you later discovered was a mistake?

_____

_____

_____

What did you do when you made the discovery?

_____

_____

_____

What does Ecclesiastes 5:6 say about what our words can do? How is that similar to what Jesus said about simply letting our yes be yes and our no be no in Matthew 5:37?

_____

_____

_____

What does the "Teacher" conclude in Ecclesiastes 5:7?

_____

_____

_____

What are we to do instead of dreaming and using "many words"?

_____

_____

_____

Now read Ecclesiastes 5:2. What does this verse tell us about our relationship to God?

_____

_____

_____

If your words are few but your actions reflect an attitude that is in awe of God, how will that impact your participation in First Place 4 Health?

_____

_____

_____

Thank You, Lord, for forgiving me when I make vows I cannot keep, especially vows that are harmful to me and damaging to my relationship with You. Amen.

REFLECTION AND APPLICATION

Day 6

Compassionate Father, it is so much easier to talk and dream than to take the action I know pleases You. Forgive me for not immediately responding to Your call. Amen.

During this week's Bible study, we have looked at the danger of making vows. List five things you have learned from this week's study about the futility of making vows.

1. _____

2. _____

3. _____

4. _____

5. _____

Ecclesiastes 5:7 tells us that "much dreaming and many words are meaningless." What dreams have you talked about but not yet put into action? (You might want to look at the list of goals and expectations you made at the beginning of this week's study as you answer this question.)

_____

_____

_____

_____

_____

_____

What do you need to do "at once" in order to turn your "dreaming" and "boasting" into an action plan that will yield results?

_____

_____

_____

_____

Are you going to immediately do what Jesus is asking you to do, or are you going to keep putting off until tomorrow what you are being asked to do today? Why, or why not?

_____

_____

_____

_____

_____

REFLECTION AND APPLICATION

*Loving Lord, how thankful I am that You see
my folly and love me anyway. Amen.*

As we have seen, one small act of obedience is more pleasing to God than gran-diose promises that never come to fruition. Rather than making impulsive vows, we are to make a plan of action and quietly obey our Master. What plans have you made that will lead to the successful accomplishment of your First Place 4 Health goals? In the space below, write your goal and then write out the daily action steps you will take to make this dream become a reality.

My First Place 4 Health vision:

_____

_____

_____

_____

Steps I will take on a daily basis to turn this vision into a reality:

_____

_____

_____

_____

Using what you have learned in this week's study, write a prayer to God in which you commit both the vision and the action steps to Him. (Remember as you write that there is a big difference between a vow and a commitment!) You might also want to record your prayer in your prayer journal.

_____

_____

_____

_____

O Lord, please hear my prayer and listen to the words I am speaking in the depth of my heart. Amen.

Group Prayer Requests

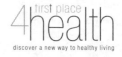

Today's Date: _____

Name	Request

Results

_____

_____

_____

_____

_____

_____

_____

Week Four

friends
and foes

Scripture Memory Verse
*Be self-controlled and alert. Your enemy the devil
prowls around like a roaring lion looking for someone to devour.*

1 Peter 5:8

In our haste to reach our goals and dreams, we often forget to include some important details in our plans for success. We are so busy eyeing the prize that we fail to notice the large pothole right beneath our feet. What are some of the potential potholes you have identified so far in this Bible study?

_____

_____

_____

_____

As you will notice, these potholes can take the form of people, places or things. Going with an eating buddy to a restaurant that serves the "to die for" chocolate cake is a combination of all three! On the other hand, going with an accountability partner to the gym for an aerobic workout combines people, places and things in a positive way. Who is one person who will support and encourage you in your efforts to honor God in all you do? How does that person provide this support and encouragement?

_____

_____

_____

_____

_____

What is one place that is detrimental to your efforts to control how much you eat? What is one place that is beneficial to your efforts in First Place 4 Health?

_____

_____

_____

What is one thing that you cannot moderate and must therefore eliminate if you are to succeed in First Place 4 Health? What is one thing you can do that will enable you to practice moderation and self-control?

_____

_____

_____

_____

Day 1   YOUR ENEMY

Lord, thank You for Your precious Word and for giving me the wisdom to distinguish between friends and foes during my First Place 4 Health journey. Amen.

In the introduction to this week's study, we looked at two different classes of people, places and things. Some were friends, while some were foes. Why do you think it is important to identify both your "friends" and your "foes" as you set your First Place 4 Health goals?

_____

_____

Our memory verse for this week tells us about a specific person who actively seeks our demise. Who is that person, and what does the possessive pronoun "your" before his name tell you?

_____

_____

_____

What else does our memory verse tell us about this enemy? There are three things listed in the second sentence of our memory verse. List them below:

1. _____

2. _____

3. _____

We are first told that our enemy the devil prowls around. When you see the word "prowl," what mental picture immediately comes to mind?

_____

_____

_____

Look up the word "prowl" in a dictionary and write the definition below.

_____

_____

_____

How did the dictionary definition confirm or contradict your understanding of the word "prowl"?

_____

_____

_____

Not only is Satan our enemy, but he is also a master of deception. Look up the verses listed below and write the disguise Satan has assumed in each instance.

Bible Verse	Description of Satan
Genesis 3:1	
John 10:10	
John 12:31	
2 Corinthians 11:13-14	
Revelation 12:9	

As you look over this list, why do you think Peter first tells us that the devil is an enemy *before* going on to describe the devil's actions?

_____

_____

_____

After looking at a few of our enemy's camouflage techniques, can you better understand the first sentence in our memory verse for Week Four? Why is it imperative that we be self-controlled and alert if we are going to succeed in our First Place 4 Health efforts?

_____

_____

_____

There is another person who is stronger than the enemy, no matter what disguise Satan is currently wearing—one who gives us daily victory and daily joy! Turn to 1 John 4:4. What does this verse tell us about God?

_____

_____

_____

Father, how thankful I am that You are on my side. You are the faithful companion who will never leave me to face my problems alone. I am truly blessed. Amen.

Day 2 — SCARE TACTICS

Gracious and loving Lord, thank You for the promises in Your Word that give me the strength and tell me how to confront my adversary, the devil. Amen.

Yesterday, we identified the three things our memory verse for Week Four tells us about the devil. After first identifying the devil as the _____ , what are the three things we are told he does?

1. _____

2. _____

3. _____

In yesterday's lesson, we mentioned that it is important for us to know that the devil is our enemy. What do you recall?

_____

_____

_____

Peter goes on to tell us that our _____ the _____ prowls around _____ a _____ _____ . What do the words "like a" tell us about the devil?

_____

_____

_____

Peter is using the example of a roaring lion, something we can see and hear in the physical realm, to illustrate a spiritual truth. Think for a moment about movies and documentaries you have seen about lions in the jungle. Why do lions roar?

_____

_____

_____

A lion roars to frighten its prey or to impress the other beasts of the forest with its power and might. How is this roaring different from a silent enemy who crouches down in the grass and then sneaks up on its unsuspecting prey, catching it unawares?

_____

_____

_____

So, while the roaring of a lion may frighten us, what other purpose does the lion's roar serve—a purpose that is beneficial to prospective prey?

_____

_____

_____

Part of using the lion's roar for our benefit is learning to recognize the warning signs and sounds so that we can respond appropriately. What form has the lion's roar taken in your life since you first began this study?

_____

_____

_____

Was this roaring voice external or within your own thoughts, or both? Explain your answer.

_____

_____

_____

How can you use the truth found in 1 John 4:4 for strength and courage when Satan comes prowling in your vicinity?

_____

_____

_____

Thank You, loving Lord, for giving me the ability to recognize my enemy, the devil, so that I am not caught off guard. Thank You for giving me an enemy that roars so that I can flee to You in safety rather than become prey. Amen.

Day 3 PRAY OR PREY

Mighty and powerful God, You are my rock and my refuge, the One I can run to when my enemy threatens to disturb my peace and security. Thank You for being my provider and my protector. Amen.

Many of the illustrations used to describe spiritual truth in the New Testament first originated in Old Testament writings. Turn to Job 1:1-12. What did Satan tell God he had been doing in verse 7?

_____

_____

How is Satan's statment like what Peter says our enemy the devil does in this week's memory verse?

_____

_____

_____

_____

What did God tell Satan in Job 1:12?

_____

_____

_____

How does this statement confirm what you learned in 1 John 4:4?

_____

_____

_____

_____

Yes, Satan can roam around. He can even roar! However, God has set a limit on what Satan can and can't do to God's people. How is this truth affirmed in 1 Corinthians 10:13?

_____

_____

_____

_____

Rather than being prey, our memory verse tells us that we can take proactive measures. What are those measures?

_____

_____

_____

_____

During our Week Three, Day Three lesson, we read about a test Peter failed because he was not self-controlled and alert. What was Peter doing instead? (You might want to read Luke 22:31-33 before answering this question.)

_____

_____

_____

How is our "boasting" like the roar of a prowling lion?

_____

_____

_____

After having learned his lesson the hard way, Peter warned others about the importance of mindfulness. Turn to 1 Peter 4:7 and complete the sentence below:

Therefore be _____ _____ and _____
so that you can _____ .

First Peter 4:7 tells us that rather than becoming prey for this roaring enemy, we can _____ . How is this truth confirmed in James 4:7-8?

_____

_____

_____

When the devil comes around, what are we to do rather than give in to fear?

_____

_____

_____

Write a prayer in your prayer journal thanking God for allowing you to draw near to Him rather than being entrapped by the enemy's wiles.

_____

_____

_____

O Lord God, I am so thankful that I can run to You when the pressures of the world leave me frightened and feeling helpless. You are my strong deliverer, no matter what the trouble may be. Amen.

A DEFEATED FOE

Merciful Savior, when You died and rose again, You defeated sin and death. Thank You for allowing me to share in Your victory. Amen.

One of the reasons Satan roars like a lion is because he knows that he has been defeated. In fulfillment of God's promise to Adam and Eve in Genesis 3:15, the seed of the woman has crushed the head of the serpent. Read Genesis 3:15 and write what God told the serpent would happen because he had deceived Eve.

_____

_____

_____

When Jesus stretched out His arms on the cross and cried, "It is finished," He had accomplished His Father's plan and purpose for the redemption of the world. When Jesus rose from the dead on the third day, Satan's head had been crushed. Satan knows he's been defeated. Christ knows Satan has been defeated. Yet because we have a hard time accepting that truth in the core of our being, Satan continues to strike at our heel—and hinders us from running the good race Christ has set before us.

Before he ascended into heaven to sit at the right hand of His Father, Jesus told His disciples to expect trouble. What other truths are contained in John 16:33? (Be sure to include Jesus' reason for telling the disciples these things.)

_____

_____

_____

Now turn in your Bible to 1 John 5:1-5. After reading these words and letting them sink into your being, rewrite what John is saying in this passage.

_____

_____

_____

What does John tell us is the secret to overcoming the world—to being victorious followers of the Risen Lord Jesus (see 1 John 5:5)?

_____

_____

_____

_____

Now refer to 1 John 2:12-14. According to these verses, who have overcome the world? What is it that these individuals possess that gives them the strength to overcome the world? Explain your answer.

_____

_____

_____

_____

How can memorizing Scripture help in your efforts to overcome the evil one? (First John 2:14 tells us this truth.)

_____

_____

_____

The book of Revelation gives us a glimpse into the end of time as we know it here on earth. What weapons did the saints in Revelation 12:11 use to overcome the great dragon?

_____

_____

_____

How do Revelation 12:11 and 1 John 5:5 tell us the same truth? What is the truth that they affirm?

_____

_____

_____

Write down some of the things God has given you the ability to overcome. Use the rest of your quiet time thanking Him for giving you victory over the evil one because of what Jesus Christ has done on your behalf. (Isaiah 53:4-6 can help you more fully understand what Jesus endured to give you peace with God.)

_____

_____

_____

_____

_____

O Lord, I am like that sheep that has gone astray. Thank You for sending Jesus to take the punishment my sin deserved so that I can have daily victory and daily joy. Amen.

STARVING SIN

Day 5

Gracious God, how foolish I am when I pray for deliverance yet run right back into harm's way. Help me to realize the consequences of my actions. Amen.

A critical strategy when trying to eliminate sinful habit patterns from our lives is to recognize our vulnerability, accept it and avoid situations and places that set us up for failure. How is this truth affirmed in this week's memory verse?

_____

_____

_____

_____

Have you ever noticed the consistency of sinning Christians? Same time, same place, same companions, same circumstances, over and over again. Go back to the list of people, places and things you wrote about in the introduction to this week's Bible study. Can you see a consistent pattern emerging between the people, places and things that continually lead you astray when it comes to eating right and exercising?

_____

_____

_____

This week's memory verse urges us to be "self controlled and alert." In First Place 4 Health, we stress the importance of mindfulness. How are these concepts one and the same thing?

_____

_____

_____

_____

What are we doing when we pray for deliverance yet run right back into the enemy's territory by being around people who are not a good influence on us, or go to places where we know we will be tempted, or choose to do things we know will lead us astray?

_____

_____

_____

What did Jesus call that kind of double-minded behavior in Matthew 4:7?

_____

_____

_____

What are some of the ways you might have "put God to the test" by your behaviors in the past?

_____

_____

_____

What does Hebrews 12:1 say we are to do with the things that entangle us and keep us from running the race set before us?

_____

_____

_____

Thinking back to your people, places and things list, what is one thing you can do this week to replace one life-destroying behavior with a life-affirming action?

_____

_____

_____

Write a prayer in your journal affirming your desire to put off the things that hinder you. Be sure to include a replacement action and explain how you will go in a different direction rather than repeat the same old destructive habits.

_____

_____

_____

Sovereign Lord, I thank You that Your mercies are new every morning and that You are moved with compassion to help me in my struggle against the forces of evil. Forgive me for those times when I have resisted You and fled instead of run to You in trust, faithfulness and love. Amen.

REFLECTION AND APPLICATION

Day
6

O Lord God, thank You that I can hide Your Word in my heart so that in times of trial I will not sin against You. Amen.

Write out our Week Four memory verse below. (You can probably write it from memory by now!)

_____

_____

_____

In this verse, Peter gives us a direct command. Underline that command. Peter then tells us why he is asking us to be self-controlled and alert. In your own words, write out the motivation for desiring to be self-controlled and alert.

_____

_____

_____

What have you learned about your enemy, the devil, during this week's Bible study that will help you resist this foe? List as many lessons as you have learned.

_____

_____

_____

_____

_____

_____

_____

What can you do today to resist the devil and stand firm in your faith? (Try to be practical, not theoretical, in your answer.)

_____

_____

_____

_____

_____

_____

Gracious God, You have given me instruction. You have equipped me with the truth of Your Word. Now, O Lord, I pray for the ability to apply these instructions to my life in meaningful ways. Amen.

Day 7 · REFLECTION AND APPLICATION

Thank You for giving me all I need to resist the devil. Thank You for sending Jesus to save me from my sins so that I can draw near to You. Amen.

Although Peter uses the example of a roaring lion to describe Satan, Solomon uses another animal to portray the work of our ancient foe. Turn in your Bible to Song of Songs 2:15. What animal is Solomon talking about in this verse?

_____

_____

_____

Imagine for a moment that your heart is a garden—a garden that is being cultivated and tilled by the Master Gardener according to His good will and pleasure. Suddenly, some cute little foxes begin to invade the Master's field and devour the budding vines before they can bear fruit. Now remember, this is not a roaring lion that will cause you great alarm. These are cute little foxes—baby foxes—something you might consider annoying but would probably be inclined to play with rather than destroy. Nevertheless, these cute little pests have the potential to devour what is precious to God. They can invade the garden of your heart, making it unfruitful.

Now give these "little foxes" descriptions that will reveal their true nature. For instance, these might be things that gobble up your time, things that sap your energy, or even things that keep you worried and awake at night—and unable to get restorative sleep. Name at least five little foxes that are nibbling away at the word of truth being planted in your heart:

1. _____
2. _____
3. _____
4. _____
5. _____

After naming them, pick one little fox you will catch and eliminate this week, and then write down how you plan to exterminate it.

_____
_____
_____
_____
_____
_____
_____

O Lord, Your divine power has given me everything I need to live a life pleasing to You. Thank You for loving me as I am—and for calling me to that place You want me to be. Amen.

Group Prayer Requests

first place
4health

Today's Date: _____

Name	Request

Results

_____
_____
_____
_____
_____
_____

our battle hymn

SCRIPTURE MEMORY VERSE
*The weapons we fight with are not the weapons of the world.
On the contrary, they have divine power to demolish strongholds.*

2 CORINTHIANS 10:4

"For though we live in the world, we do not wage war as the world does," the apostle Paul declares in 2 Corinthians 10:3. As Christ followers, we are called to live in peace—and to wage war. We are to live in peace with God, peace with self and peace with our brothers and sisters in Christ, but war against the forces of evil that threaten that peace.

If those forces were as obvious as the roaring lion we learned about in last week's lessons, or even as visible as the little foxes that destroy what God has planted in our hearts, the battle we wage would be easy to fight. But Scripture is very clear: the enemy we fight against is not part of the physical realm, not comprised of flesh and blood. Listen to Paul's words to the Ephesians:

> For our struggle is not against flesh and blood, but against the rulers, against the authorities, against the powers of this dark world and against the spiritual forces of evil in the heavenly realms (Ephesians 6:12).

As we begin this week's lesson, spend a few moments reflecting on the apostle Paul's words. After you have done so, summarize what Paul is saying in your own voice. Pay special attention to how Paul describes the enemy we battle and where that enemy is located.

REPENTANCE AND REST, QUIETNESS AND TRUST

Merciful Savior, keep me from evil today. When I am weak, give me strength. When I am tempted, grant me courage. When I am disheartened, give me hope. Amen.

If we were called to contend against a visible enemy, we could arm ourselves with the best weaponry that modern technology could devise. We could attend a prestigious military academy and study advanced battlefield tactics. We could employ armored tanks and artillery and march into battle with confidence in our superior equipment and military prowess. But throughout the pages of Scripture, we see the futility of depending on human strength.

Turn to Isaiah 30:15-18 and read what the Sovereign Lord tells His people about depending on the world's might and power. Then, in the table below list God's way of fighting this spiritual battle versus man's way of trying to overcome our ancient foe. ("Swift horses" in this passage represent the world's dependence on might to solve conflict, so list the things we depend on in our modern world as you complete this exercise.)

God's Way of Fighting	Man's Way of Fighting

How can repentance, rest, quietness and trust become part of the divine weaponry you employ in your First Place 4 Health endeavors (see Isaiah 30:15)?

_____

_____

_____

What component of the First Place 4 Health program is about repentance, rest, quietness and trust?

_____

_____

_____

Have you been consistent in spending quiet time with God each day as part of your ongoing battle against the forces of evil? Why or why not?

_____

_____

_____

List several things you can eliminate from your schedule so that you can spend more time with your Lord, the One who is the source of your joy and strength.

_____

_____

_____

_____

_____

O Lord God, the weapons You tell me to use are indeed contrary to the world's ways. Help me to sit before You in quietness and trust rather than depending on displays of might and power that are useless in this battle I fight daily. Amen.

THE JOY OF THE LORD

Day 2

O Lord God, when I am afraid, I will trust in You. When I feel like running away from my problems, I will sit quietly and wait for You to come to my assistance. Amen.

Our Week Five memory verse tells us an important truth about the daily battle we wage against the forces that seek our demise. Write those words of truth:

_____

_____

_____

These words give us some important information about our spiritual weapons. Summarize what 2 Corinthians 10:4 teaches us about the weapons we fight with.

_____

_____

_____

Yesterday, we learned about four of the divine weapons we are called to employ in the battle against evil. List those four weapons:

1. _____

2. _____

3. _____

4. _____

How are these four divine weapons different from the weapons that the world relies on?

_____

_____

_____

The last of the divine weapons listed in Isaiah 30:15 is "trust." But exactly who is it that we are to trust in, and why? Turn to Proverbs 3:5-8 and carefully read these words before answering this question.

_____

_____

_____

_____

How is trusting in the Lord with all your heart different from relying on your own understanding when it comes to fighting a spiritual battle?

_____

_____

_____

_____

In 2 Chronicles 20, we read about another divine weapon tactic that we can employ. The people of Israel were facing a fierce and mighty foe. From a human perspective, God's people were ill equipped and outnumbered. Yet as the enemy forces marched toward the Israelites, Jehoshaphat called on them to put their trust in God in a very tangible way. Turn to 2 Chronicles 20:20-22 and read what the Israelites did. What did you learn from reading these words?

_____

_____

_____

_____

How can you begin to use each of these as your divine weapons?

_____

_____

_____

_____

Nehemiah tells us that the joy of the Lord is our strength (see Nehemiah 8:10). The apostle Paul tells us that we can rejoice always because the Lord is near (see Philippians 4:4-5). How is joy in the Lord, as shown by praise, thanksgiving and rejoicing, part of your First Place 4 Health program?

_____

_____

_____

_____

How is praising God in the midst of adversity different from giving in to doubt and fear when the forces of evil threaten our peace and security?

_____

_____

_____

_____

Spend some time praising God now. Perhaps you would like to use the words of 2 Chronicles 20:21 as a way of remembering that God's incredible love for you endures forever.

How good it is to trust You, O Lord God Almighty! Today I will rejoice in all my circumstances because I know that You are near. Amen.

THE ARMOR OF GOD

I love You, O Lord, my strength. On my own, I can do no good thing. Yet in Your strength and might I can do all You ask of me. Thank You! Amen.

Our memory verse for this week tells us that the weapons we fight with are different from the weapons the world employs. In fact, our weapons are not only different, but they are also contrary to the world's way and opposed to people's natural way of thinking and reasoning.

Review the words we read in Ephesians 6:12 in the introduction to this week's Bible study and your reflections on the enemy we fight against. As you read, ask God to give you spiritual eyes to see new insights. What new understanding of this verse did the Holy Spirit illuminate for you as you read it today?

Ephesians 6:10-11 gives us information about where the power to fight this spiritual battle comes from. According to Ephesians 6:10, where does our strength come from?

How is this truth affirmed in David's words in Psalm 121:2-4?

Before you continue with today's study, thank the Lord for watching over you day and night and giving you the strength to live a life pleasing to Him.

Go back to Ephesians 6:13-18 and begin to look at Paul's description of the divine weapons that God supplies for our daily use. Paul calls it the "full armor of God." In verses 14-18, Paul lists seven divine weapons. List each of these in the table below, and then in the column beside each piece of spiritual armor, write the opposite weaponry that the world uses in battle. For instance, instead of truth, the way of the world is deception, denial, duplicity and lies.

God's Armor	The World's Battle Gear
Truth	*Deception, denial, duplicity and lies*

When you are finished, review the list and identify one piece of God's armor you can put on today that will help you in your First Place 4 Health efforts. What is the piece of armor you need most right now, and how can you use it to overcome the forces of evil that keep you from being strong in God's power?

_____

_____

_____

Next, identify an area where you have relied on the world's philosophies and psychology in a vain attempt to overcome the spiritual forces that wage war against your soul. Repentance is another of our spiritual weapons, so confess your failings to God and determine how to fight this spiritual battle a better way—His way—from now on. (You might want to record your thoughts in your prayer journal for privacy.)

_____

_____

_____

Finally, think about some of the other spiritual weapons we learned about last week and write down how you will use those weapons in your First Place 4

Health efforts. Rest in God's presence as you allow His might and power to be your source of strength.

You, O Lord God, are the One who trains my hands and my mind for battle. I can do all things, including overcoming the forces of evil, because I trust in You as my source and supply. Amen.

Day
4

A DOUBLE-EDGED SWORD

Gracious God, You have given me Your Spirit and Your Word. Help me to allow the Spirit to apply Your truth to my life in meaningful ways. Amen.

Yesterday, we spent time studying Paul's words in Ephesians 6:10-18. What spiritual weapon did you decide to employ in your fight against Satan's schemes?

_____

_____

_____

How have you put that choice into action since doing that lesson?

_____

_____

_____

One of the pieces of weaponry Paul lists is "the sword of the Spirit." According to Ephesians 6:17, what is the sword of the Spirit?

_____

_____

_____

We are given some additional information about the sword of the Spirit in the book of Revelation. Turn to Revelation 1:16 and record how the sword is described in that verse.

_____

_____

_____

Hebrews 4:12-13 gives us even more information about the sword of the Spirit as part of our spiritual arsenal. What new things did you learn about the Word of God from this passage?

_____

_____

_____

The sword of the Spirit is not only double-edged but also living and active. What does that tell you about God's Word?

_____

_____

_____

For God's Word to be living and active in your battle against the spiritual forces of evil, what must you do?

_____

_____

_____

If your Bible sits unread on a shelf, collecting dust rather than imparting power, is it living and active in your life? Why or why not?

_____

_____

_____

Hebrews 4:12 tells us that the Word of God penetrates our being to allow us to separate ourselves from those things that keep us from living a life pleasing to God. In order for the Word of God to penetrate your being, what must you do? (In answering this question, please remember that our Lord gave us free will and therefore will not force us to accept His truth.)

_____

_____

_____

_____

Have you opened your heart and mind to receive the truth of God's Word so that it can replace the faulty messages that play in your mind? Your *First Place 4 Health Member's Guide* contains several worksheets designed to help you replace Satan's lies with the truth of God's Word (see pages 43-68). If you have not already done these worksheets, set aside some time to complete them.

Hebrews 4:12 goes on to tell us that in addition to penetrating our inner being, dividing soul and spirit, joints and marrow, the Word of God has another important function. What does the Word do to our thoughts and attitudes?

_____

_____

_____

What mental thought or attitude of the heart do you need to submit to the Word of God so that you can stand strong in your faith when threatened by that roaring lion we learned about in previous lessons?

_____

_____

_____

Find a truth from God's Word that you can use to transform that thought or attitude and write it below. You can be part of the transformation process by reading that verse or passage from Scripture each time negative thoughts and attitudes start to flood your mind and heart.

_____

_____

_____

Hebrews 4:13 ends with a sobering thought: "Everything is uncovered and laid bare before the eyes of him to whom we must give account." If the Lord were standing before you right now, what inner thoughts and attitudes would be uncovered and laid bare?

_____

_____

_____

Confess those failings and faults to God in prayer so that you can receive mercy and grace from your compassionate and forgiving Lord. Write this confession below or in your prayer journal.

_____

_____

_____

_____

_____

Gracious God, Your compassion and mercy are beyond my comprehension. I am grateful that You are a God who forgives my sins and removes the burden of my guilt in Christ Jesus my Lord. Amen.

THE POWER OF PRAYER   Day 5

O Lord, Your Word is a lamp to my feet and a light to my path.
Today I pray for grace to receive Your truth in faith and love and strength
to follow on the path You've set before me. Amen.

As we begin today's lesson, reread Ephesians 6:10-18 and ask the Lord to illuminate anything in this passage He knows you need to understand more clearly. Each time we read God's Word, He will reveal new truths to us if we will allow Him to show us exciting new things in old familiar passages.

What new thing did God bring to your awareness as you reread this passage?

_____

_____

_____

Notice that Paul lists the first six pieces of spiritual armor in verses 14-17. Yet the final piece of armor is contained in a longer verse. What is the piece of spiritual armor listed in verse 18, and why do you think Paul gives this spiritual weaponry more attention?

_____

_____

_____

When trials, temptations and other troubles come, the world swings into action. When the going gets tough, the tough go shopping, start eating, begin raging, wring their hands in worry, blame others, or try to outrun the foe. But Christians do it differently. We drop to our knees in prayer! Think about those two opposite ways of handling the stress of life and write about how these two battle tactics are contrary to one another.

_____

_____

_____

_____

_____

When and where does Ephesians 6:18 tell us we should pray?

And pray in the Spirit on _____ _____ with _____ _____ of _____ and _____ .

What does the presence of the word "all" tell you?

_____

_____

_____

According to Ephesians 6:18, is there any time or place we are not to pray?

_____

_____

_____

Paul also tells us to be alert. How does this correspond with Peter's words in our Week Four memory verse?

_____

_____

_____

_____

Recall from last week's lesson what Peter said in 1 Peter 4:7, the reason we are to remain clear minded and alert. Write that reason below in your own words.

_____

_____

_____

Look back at the paragraph that describes how the world handles trial, temptation and trouble. Are these actions part of being clear-minded and alert?

_____

_____

_____

How is prayer part of the spiritual weaponry we learned about in the Isaiah 30:15 passage we studied in Day One?

_____

_____

_____

In Isaiah 30:15, we are given four characteristics of effective prayer. What are those four elements?

1. _____

2. _____

3. _____

4. _____

Do your prayers include these four components? If not, what element do you need to add today so that you can fully utilize the power of prayer in your battle against the spiritual forces of evil?

_____

_____

_____

_____

Having identified the deficiency in your prayer life, what action steps will you take today to put on the whole armor of God when it comes to prayer?

_____

_____

_____

Sovereign Lord, how grateful I am for the awesome power of prayer. Please forgive me for the times I have rushed into action rather than humbling myself before You and dropping to my knees in prayer. Amen.

Day 6

REFLECTION AND APPLICATION

Loving Lord, I know the world's weapons are not effective in fighting spiritual battles. Help me to learn and apply the truth of Your Word so that I am equipped for the daily battle as I fight against the spiritual forces of evil. Amen.

Write this week's memory verse from memory in the space below. After writing the verse, underline the words "divine power." Why is divine power the only way to overcome the spiritual forces of evil?

_____

_____

_____

Now draw a circle around the word "strongholds." When we use this word in the context of this week's memory verse, it is a negative force that keeps us from making spiritual progress. However, the Bible uses this word in another way that is vital to our First Place 4 Health program. Look up the following verses to learn about this other type of stronghold:

2 Samuel 22:3: _____

_____

_____

Psalm 9:9: _____

_____

_____

Psalm 18:2: _____

_____

_____

Psalm 27:1: _____

_____

_____

Psalm 144:2: _____

_____

_____

What did you learn about the word "stronghold" from these verses?

_____

_____

_____

_____

On this day of reflection and application, spend some time contemplating how you can use the word "stronghold" as a spiritual weapon against the "strongholds" that must be destroyed if you are to succeed in your First Place 4 Health endeavors. In completing this exercise, you will need to draw from all the material you learned this week—all the weapons in your spiritual arsenal. Write your thoughts below or in your journal.

_____

_____

_____

_____

_____

_____

Lord, You are my stronghold and the source of my strength. When I cling to You, I am given the power to overcome the wiles of the enemy. Amen.

REFLECTION AND APPLICATION

Loving God, You are my fortress, my stronghold and my deliverer, my shield in whom I take refuge (see Psalm 144:2). Amen.

This week, we have learned about spiritual weapons with divine power. Today, we will review the spiritual weaponry we have added to our spiritual arsenal. In the table below, begin an inventory of the weapons that you have learned about this week. Next to each item, list the way you will apply this particular weapon to the battle you are waging as you travel toward health, wholeness and a lifestyle that is pleasing to God. List at least seven weapons and their applications.

Spiritual Weapon with Divine Power	First Place 4 Health Application

Thank You, gracious Lord, for preparing and equipping me to overcome the strongholds that block my ability to make forward progress in First Place 4 Health. You are my strength and my shield, the One I can run to when the battle is fierce and I am in need of comfort and safety. Amen.

Group Prayer Requests

4 first place
health

Today's Date: _____

Name	Request

Results

_____

_____

_____

_____

_____

_____

_____

pave the pathway with prayer

SCRIPTURE MEMORY VERSE

Call to me and I will answer you and tell you great and unsearchable things you do not know.

JEREMIAH 33:3

Last week, we learned about some of the divine-power weapons we can use in our fight against the spiritual forces of evil. We also learned about two types of reactions to the stress and trials of life: (1) the reaction the world makes when faced with trouble, and (2) the reaction that we are called to make when the pressures of the world are too heavy to bear.

In addition to being part of our spiritual weaponry, prayer is the source of wisdom and strength. When we call on God, He promises to give us wisdom and knowledge that the world cannot comprehend. Our memory verse for Week Six comes from Jeremiah 33. At the time these words were written, Jeremiah was in prison, and Jerusalem was under siege. Yet even in this desperate situation, the Lord gave Jeremiah words of encouragement and hope.

Turn to Jeremiah 33:10-16 and read God's powerful words to the imprisoned prophet. What situation in your life currently seems desolate and without hope?

_____

_____

_____

How can you apply the Lord's words to the problems that plague your life?

_____

_____

_____

Our God is a God of hope and encouragement who sends us His Word to fill us with strength, courage and hope. Take heart! No matter how dark the night, our Lord promises to bring restoration. He will light a path for us if we will only trust in Him and listen to His words.

CALL ON ME

Lord God, You invite me to call on You at all times and in all circumstances.
Thank You for inviting me into Your awesome presence! Amen.

Throughout the history of salvation, our gracious God has invited His people to call on Him—and saints throughout the ages have responded to that invitation by calling on the name of the Lord their God. And while we think that calling on the name of the Lord is something we do only when we are in distress, Scripture gives us many examples of God's people calling on Him when they were not in imminent danger.

Look up the three verses listed below and describe why God's people called on Him for each verse.

1 Chronicles 16:8-12: _____

_____

_____

Psalm 105:1-3: _____

_____

_____

Isaiah 12:1-6: _____

_____

What do these verses tell you about the importance of calling on God when you are rejoicing and remembering the good things He has done for you?

_____

_____

_____

Recall from our Week Five story what happened to Jehoshaphat and God's people when they marched into battle praising God. (If you need to refresh your memory, reread 2 Chronicles 20:20-22.) Since reading that account last week, what have you done to incorporate the spiritual weapon of praise into your First Place 4 Health program?

_____

_____

_____

_____

When Peter addressed the crowd on Pentecost, he quoted the prophet Joel as part of his explanation of what was happening that day. Turn to Acts 2:14-21 and read Peter's words. What is the promise contained in Acts 2:21?

_____

_____

_____

_____

Have you called on the name of the Lord, asking Him to forgive your sins and become the Lord of your life? Why or why not?

_____

_____

_____

_____

If you answered "yes" to that question, spend time praising God for the marvelous gift of salvation! If you have not called on the Lord and asked Him to be your Savior, please talk to your First Place 4 Health group leader, your pastor or a mature Christian friend. Your *First Place 4 Health Member's Guide* has more information on your new life in Christ. Please take the time to read it now!

Thank You, gracious and merciful Lord, that when I call on You I am assured that You will answer me. With You as the Lord of my life, I know that I can receive grace and help in my time of need. Amen.

THEY CALLED, GOD SAVED

*O Lord God, You lift the needy out of their affliction. How good
it is to consider Your great love for those in distress. Amen.*

Psalm 107 is an epic-type poem that tells us about the distress of several different groups of people that each had one thing in common. Read Psalm 107:1-32 and list the four groups described in the chart below. Next to each group, list what they did that aroused God's compassion. In the third column, list what God did for them in response to their pleas.

Group	What Action They Took	How God Responded

Look back at your summary. Is there one particular group you can identify with more than the other? Which one, and why?

_____

_____

_____

Psalm 107:20 tells of a specific action that God took on behalf of those who suffered affliction because of their rebellious ways. What was that action?

_____

_____

_____

Think of a recent time when you were in distress and called God for help. How was God's Word an integral part of the solution that brought you help and healing? How did it free you from the things that kept you in distress and despair?

_____

_____

_____

Look at Psalm 107:23-28. Was God's response to the people in these verses contingent upon the reason for their affliction?

_____

_____

_____

What does the fact that God rescued both the innocent victims and those who were in a predicament because of their rebellious actions tell you?

_____

_____

_____

It is the cries of God's people that evoke His response, not the reason for the situation they find themselves in! What an amazing God we serve! Write a prayer of thanksgiving below or in your prayer journal. Begin your prayer with the words from Psalm 107:1: "Give thanks to the Lord, for he is good; his love endures forever."

_____

_____

_____

_____

_____

_____

O Lord, You are good, and You are loving. How fortunate I am to be the recipient of Your mercy, grace and love. Amen.

AN ANSWER HAS BEEN GIVEN

Day 3

Hear my prayer, O Lord, and listen to the voice of my supplication. You are the giver of all good gifts and the source of all wisdom. O Lord, hear and answer, for I am in need of Your healing touch. Amen.

Daniel was a prophet who called on the name of the Lord God many times during his long and eventful life. On one such occasion, Daniel was saved from the hungry lions because of his faith and trust in God's provision and protection. (Ironically, Daniel was thrown into the lion's den for praying!)

On one occasion, Daniel was praying for the restoration of the city of Jerusalem. Read what happened as a result of Daniel's prayers in Daniel 9:20-23. How are Gabriel's words to Daniel similar to our memory verse for this week?

_____

_____

_____

_____

As a result of Daniel's prayers, he was given insight and understanding. What particular problem or situation do you need insight and understanding about right now? Have you called on the name of the Lord in anticipation of receiving the wisdom you seek? Why, or why not?

_____

_____

_____

Gabriel told Daniel that as soon as he began to pray, an answer had been given. Spiritual forces had been set in motion that would result in the very thing for which he was praying. But restoration took more than 70 years. During the waiting time, Israel learned many more painful lessons, yet Daniel was confident that his prayers had been heard and an answer had been given. What does this teach you about the importance of persistence in prayer?

_____

_____

_____

Think of a time you prayed for restoration and healing, especially as it applied to weight loss and physical fitness. Did you wait for God's response, confident that an answer had been given, or did you give up and go in another direction?

_____

_____

_____

Many of us remember a time when we went to an authority figure asking for help or advice only to be scolded and ridiculed. Turn in your Bible to James 1:5 to see how God treats those who come to Him asking for advice or wisdom. What did you discover?

_____

_____

_____

James 1:6 tells us how we are to act when we come to God in prayer. What does this verse say?

_____

_____

_____

Recall a time when you prayed for wisdom about your personal wellness concerns and then continued to eat to excess or not exercise. According to James 1:6, what were you doing?

_____

_____

_____

What truth does James 1:7 give us about those who are "double-minded"?

_____

_____

_____

What are you really doing when you focus on just one aspect of your four-sided being but neglect one or more of the others?

_____

_____

_____

What are some ways that you use prayer to add stability and balance to your First Place 4 Health endeavors?

_____

_____

_____

_____

_____

_____

Compassionate Father, how thankful I am that I can come to You in confidence that You will not scold or ridicule me. Instead of chiding me, You promise to give me the wisdom I seek. Thank You. Amen.

GREAT AND UNSEARCHABLE THINGS — Day 4

Lord, thank You for the presence of the Holy Spirit in my life. Open my heart and teach me the things that You want me to know. Amen.

Our memory verse contains a word we don't often use: "unsearchable." Write out Jeremiah 33:3, and then circle that word.

_____

_____

_____

Now, look up the word "unsearchable" in a college-level dictionary. Write out the definitions you discover.

_____

_____

Using the definition that you think best captures the essence of Jeremiah 33:3, insert that alternate word into the memory verse you just wrote out. Does that make the meaning of this week's memory verse clearer?

_____

_____

_____

_____

Our memory verse from Week Two is part of the instruction Moses gave the Israelites just before they were to cross into the Promised Land. If you can, write out Deuteronomy 30:11 from memory, or look at the verse to refresh your memory and then write it down.

_____

_____

_____

_____

Through Moses, God told the people that what He was asking of them was not beyond their reach. Then, in anticipation of the people's grumbling and complaining, He gave them some examples of where His Word was *not* to be found. Read Deuteronomy 30:12-13 and write what God told the Israelites.

_____

_____

_____

_____

After telling the people where His Word was not, God told them where it could be found. According to Deuteronomy 30:14, where is the Word the people are to obey?

_____

_____

_____

_____

Before Jesus was crucified, He consoled His grieving disciples by telling them about One who would take His place and remind them of what He had said to them while He was still among them. Look at John 14:26. Who is this person?

_____

_____

_____

How do the words of John 14:26 correspond with this week's memory verse?

_____

_____

_____

What truth has the Holy Spirit brought to your awareness during today's study?

_____

_____

_____

How do you intend to respond to the Spirit's gentle reminder?

_____

_____

_____

_____

_____

Lord God, You do not leave me to face my problems alone. Your words are in my mouth and in my heart. I have no excuse for not obeying You. Amen.

OVERLOOKING GOD'S ANSWER

Day
5

Lord, help me to thank You for the little things You do for me each day. Amen.

Although our God is always faithful to hear and answer our prayers, we are not always quick to see the answer He provides. The Bible gives us a wonderful story to illustrate how we often overlook the very answer we are praying for. Turn in your Bible to Acts 12 and read verses 1-16.

After reading the story, write your version of the events being told in this passage as if you were an on-the-spot reporter giving an account to the news media.

_____

_____

_____

Who was the first person in the story who did not believe God had heard and answered the people's prayers for Peter's deliverance?

_____

_____

_____

Rather than rejoicing in his miraculous escape from prison, what did Peter think was happening?

_____

_____

_____

What happened when Peter finally came to his senses? What did he do?

_____

_____

_____

What were the people inside the house doing as Peter stood outside knocking?

_____

_____

_____

Rhoda, the servant girl, recognized Peter's voice. But in her excitement, what did she fail to do?

_____

_____

How did those praying for Peter's deliverance react to Rhoda's words?

_____

_____

_____

Recall a time in your life when you were praying for a miracle but didn't recognize God's hand bringing deliverance until after the fact. What did you do when you came to your senses?

_____

_____

_____

How did the others who had been praying with you and for you respond when the answer came? Were they doubtful, happy, jealous, afraid or astonished?

_____

_____

_____

Peter continued to knock on the door until they let him in. How have you continued to witness to God's deliverance even in the midst of naysayers and doubters who think God's miraculous answer is too good to be true?

_____

_____

_____

How have you been a faithful witness to the deliverance you have experienced in the First Place 4 Health program?

_____

_____

_____

Like Peter, are you the first one to overlook what God is doing in your life, thinking the events are just "coincidence"? Explain your answer.

_____

_____

_____

When others doubt the miraculous way that God is working in your life, do you continue to give Him all the praise and glory? Why or why not?

_____

_____

_____

What have you learned about the importance of prayer—and believing your prayers will be answered—from reading the story of Peter's miraculous escape from prison?

_____

_____

_____

Forgive me, Father, for the times I see Your miracle-in-the-making but fail to recognize Your hand in the events that are bringing forth my deliverance. Amen.

Day
6

REFLECTION AND APPLICATION

Gracious God, You lead me, guide me and teach me the way I should go. Thank You for sending the Holy Spirit to guide me into all truth. Amen.

During the past five weeks, you have learned many lessons and have been challenged to apply those lessons to your life. Today is an opportunity to reflect on what you have learned and how you have been able to use that information in a positive way. The table on the following page will allow you to recall what the Holy Spirit has brought to your attention so far during this session. Hopefully, you have learned many things each week, so pick the one teaching lesson that you feel is most important to your First Place 4 Health success. Next to that major lesson learned, write how you have applied that lesson in ways that are producing transformation.

Week	Most Important Lesson	Application to Your Life
Two		
Three		
Four		
Five		
Six		

Now summarize the progress that you have made so far in this session of First Place 4 Health.

_____

_____

_____

_____

Spend the rest of your quiet time praising God for the lessons you have learned and the progress you have made. If you choose to write your prayer of thanksgiving, please do so in the space below or use your prayer journal.

_____

_____

_____

_____

_____

You, O Lord, have done marvelous things for me, and I am filled with joy. Amen.

Day 7 | REFLECTION AND APPLICATION

It is good to praise Your name, O Lord Most High. Amen.

After five weeks of doing written exercises, it is time to put on our walking shoes for a different type of exercise! Throughout our study, we have seen God's people using the words, "Give thanks to the Lord, for He is good. His love endures forever." Practice saying this verse a few times to get comfortable with the cadence. Now go for a walk and use these words as your Battle Hymn. As you walk and repeat these words, remember how the Israelites walked into battle saying these very words. Recall the good things the Lord has done for you. Thank Him for freeing you from the bondage of overeating and not taking care of yourself. This is prayer in motion—a prayer that honors the Creator who gave you a wonderfully made body to enjoy while you are here on earth.

Thank You, Gracious God, for allowing me to live and move and have my being in You. Amen.

Group Prayer Requests

first place
4health

Today's Date: _____

Name	Request

Results

_____

_____

_____

_____

_____

_____

_____

living a life
pleasing to God

SCRIPTURE MEMORY VERSE
We make it our goal to please him,
whether we are at home in the body or away from it.
2 CORINTHIANS 5:9

We have reached the midpoint of this session of First Place 4 Health! If you have been diligent in your efforts, you should be seeing subtle changes that herald a new beginning—physical, mental, emotional and spiritual progress that tell you that your diligent effort has not been in vain.

One of the promises God gives us is that we will reap what we sow: "Remember this: Whoever sows sparingly also reaps sparingly, and whoever sows generously will also reap generously" (2 Corinthians 9:6). You can be assured that if you have been earnestly seeking God by keeping Him first in all things, you will reap the results in proportion to your efforts.

Before moving forward to the second half of our Bible study, it is time to rest and reflect on the progress you have made during the first five weeks—to make an honest assessment of your growth in grace and knowledge. In the introduction to the Week Three portion of this Bible study, you were asked to envision what you hoped to accomplish during this session of First Place 4 Health. Your self-assessment was not just about physical improvement; it also included the other aspects of your four-sided being. Turn back to that assessment and review what you wrote. Now look at those four areas again and record the prog-ress you have made in each area:

Physically: _____

_____

_____

Mentally: _____

_____

_____

Emotionally: _____

_____

_____

Spiritually: _____

_____

_____

What did this assessment reveal about the way you are managing your efforts?

_____

_____

_____

Be sure to give God the glory, honor and praise in the areas in which you see improvement. In the areas where you have not been diligent, determine to do things differently from now on. The Lord's mercies are new every morning. Praise God, each day can be a new beginning in First Place 4 Health!

PLEASING GOD

Day
1

May the words of my mouth and the meditation of my heart be pleasing in Your sight, O Lord, my Rock and my Redeemer. Amen (see Psalm 19:14).

Our memory verse for Week Seven tells us a vital truth: No matter what other goals we might have in First Place 4 Health, our primary goal—the one that supersedes all others—is to please God! But in order to accomplish that goal, we must learn what pleases Him. His ways are not our ways, and His thoughts are not our thoughts. Our best efforts apart from doing what pleases Him are futile. Perhaps that is why the apostle Paul continually urged his readers to find out what is pleasing to the Lord (see Ephesians 5:10).

All healthy relationships are based on honest, open communication, and so it is with our relationship with God. He does not expect us to guess about what pleases Him or to tiptoe around trying to figure out His moods and desires. God is not a dysfunctional communicator who expects us to read His mind! He clearly tells us in His Word what pleases Him.

As in all things, our example for making it our goal to please God comes from Jesus, the One who came to show us the way to the Father. Look up the following passages in your Bible, recording what you discover beside each verse:

John 4:34: _____

_____

John 5:30: _____

_____

John 6:38: _____

_____

John 8:29: _____

_____

Based on what you read in these verses, is there a difference between doing God's revealed will and doing what pleases God?

_____

_____

_____

Yes, doing God's will and pleasing Him are synonymous. Living in purposeful obedience to God's revealed will is what pleases Him! How can you apply this truth to your First Place 4 Health endeavors?

_____

_____

_____

_____

Lord God, thank You for Jesus, the author and perfecter of my faith. He came to show me how to live a life pleasing to You. Help me to always follow His example. Amen.

WE MAKE IT OUR GOAL

Day 2

Faithful Father, You have promised to show me the way and guide me on straight paths. Help me to discern Your good, pleasing and perfect will for my life. Amen.

One of the principles of setting goals is to make the end we strive for specific. It is one thing to say we want to please God, but it is another to know the specific things we must do if we are to achieve that goal. On a human level, we have all been in relationships in which pleasing the other party was an impossible dream—or in which we had to continually guess what the other person wanted from us. Not so with God! As we learned in yesterday's lesson, God is the perfect communicator. He desires that we know Him. He longs to tell us what is pleasing to Him and asks that we read His Word so that we can discern His will.

Our God delights in our purposeful obedience and grieves when we ignore Him. "If my people would but listen to me, if Israel would follow my ways, how quickly would I subdue their enemies and turn my hand against their foes," the Lord declared in Psalm 81:13. For those of us trying to overcome negative habit patterns, that is an awesome promise! Listening to God and discerning what pleases Him is not just a noble goal but also essential to our success!

On the chart below are some specific things that God tells us please Him. Beside each verse, write the action that pleases God. Then, in the third column, write one thing you can do today to incorporate that action into your First Place 4 Health program.

Scripture Verse	Action that Pleases God	First Place 4 Health Application
Psalm 51:16-17		
Psalm 69:31		
Proverbs 15:8		

Scripture Verse	Action that Pleases God	First Place 4 Health Application
Micah 6:8		
Romans 12:1		
Galatians 6:7-8		
Hebrews 11:6		

One of the ways we become aware of what pleases God is to keep a record of the verses, like those listed above, that tell us what God desires of us. Your journal is an excellent place to keep this list.

Your desire, O Lord, is that I keep You first in all things. Help me to learn what specific actions I must choose in order to please You. Amen.

Day 3

DETESTABLE IN HIS SIGHT

Prepare my heart, O God, to accept Your Word. Silence in me any voices but Your own so that I may hear Your Word and obey it. Amen.

Just as our gracious God clearly tells us what pleases Him, He is also specific about the things He detests. Proverbs 6:16-19 gives us a list of seven things that are detestable in the Lord's sight. Turn to that passage and write down the seven detestable things listed in those verses:

1. _____

2. _____

3. _____

4. _____

5. _____

6. _____

7. _____

Two of these "detestable things" are worthy of special attention: (1) haughty eyes, and (2) feet that are quick to rush into evil. "Haughty" is not a word we use a lot in modern-day language, so we need to be clear on the meaning of this word. Look up the word "haughty" in a dictionary and record what you find.

_____

_____

_____

Now turn to 1 Peter 5:5 and read what Peter tells us about being proud (which is another word for "haughty").

_____

_____

_____

God opposes the proud! Romans 8:31 tells us, "If God is for us, who can be against us?" Conversely, if God is opposed to us, how can we possibly succeed? How might "haughty eyes"—being proud and unteachable—keep you from succeeding in your First Place 4 Health endeavors?

_____

_____

What can you do today to humble yourself under God's mighty hand so that you can be a recipient of His favor?

_____

_____

_____

"Feet that are quick to rush into evil" is the second detestable thing we need to examine. Impulsivity is the downfall of those who seek to live a life pleasing to God. Turn in your Bible to Proverbs 4:26-27. What does God tell us to do?

_____

_____

_____

Stop and consider if you are doing anything that is keeping you from reaching your First Place 4 Health efforts. For example, if you have determined to eat nutritious foods that fuel and restore your body but are taking a path that leads you by the donut shop each day, that choice is not bringing you closer to your goals. Write down any area in which you are not taking "level paths."

_____

_____

_____

Turn to 1 John 2:15-17. What are God's instructions in this passage?

_____

_____

_____

Look again at the list of seven things in Proverbs 6:16-19 that are detestable to the Lord and pick one item that you need to eliminate from your behavior today. Next, choose a life-affirming action—a behavior that is pleasing to God—and work to feed what is good and starve what is not. Write down the behavior that you will eliminate and your action plan for accomplishing this.

_____

_____

_____

_____

You might want to call someone in your First Place 4 Health group and tell them of your plan so that they can hold you accountable to that decision.

Forgive me, compassionate Father, when my feet are quick to rush into evil. Pleasing You is my desire. Help my behavior match my words and my goals. Amen.

HOME IN THE BODY—OR AWAY FROM IT

Day
4

God, You promised to give me clarity and understanding when I ask for wisdom. Today, that is my prayer. Open my eyes to see the truth in Your Word. Amen.

We are in Day Four of our study, and by now you can probably write this week's memory verse from memory. As you write it below, meditate on what the words are saying, paying particular attention to the last part of the verse.

_____

_____

_____

When we look at this verse in the context in which it is written, we discover that the apostle Paul is talking about His desire to be away from the body and at home with the Lord. That should be the longing and goal for each of us who confess the name of Jesus as our Lord and Savior.

However, there is still rich application in the last part of our memory verse if we consider the "body" that Paul is talking about to be the Body of Christ. As Christ followers, we need to make it our goal to please God—whether we are with others who comprise the Body of Christ or are away from them. We can't live one life while in church and another when we are in the world. When our desire is to truly please God, we will live lives of integrity 24 hours a day, 7 days a week.

Acts 5 contains a well-known story about two people who tried to impress the Body but ended up offending the Lord. In order to fully understand what happened that one fateful day, we need to begin our reading in Acts 4:36 and continue through Acts 5:4. Please read that passage and then answer the following questions:

What did Barnabas, the great encourager, do that was noteworthy?

_____

_____

_____

_____

When Ananias saw the praise that Barnabas received for his actions, what did he decide to do?

_____

_____

_____

Why do you think Luke specifically tells us that his wife, Sapphira, knew about (and approved of) Ananias's scheme?

_____

_____

_____

What did Peter say to Ananias when he discovered that Ananias and his wife had kept some of the money for themselves?

_____

_____

_____

In Acts 5:4, Peter states it was not the fact that Ananias kept part of the money that was the problem. What had Ananias done to bring judgment on himself?

_____

_____

_____

Notice that Peter did not say that Ananias had lied to the believers. Whom does Peter say Ananias lied to in Acts 5:4? Why did Peter make this statement?

_____

_____

_____

How can you apply what you have just read to your First Place 4 Health efforts?

_____

_____

_____

Why is it crucial to be faithful to your desire to live for the Lord all week and be honest about your successes and failures? What is the danger in exaggerating your achievements in order to impress others in your group?

_____

_____

_____

What does James 5:16 say is a better way to handle our failures?

_____

_____

_____

How will what you learned today have an impact on your participation in First Place 4 Health?

_____

_____

_____

_____

Lord, You tell me that what I have done for other believers, I have also done for You. How often I pride myself in my humanitarian accomplishments without realizing that when I treat others wrongly, I also offend You. Please forgive me. Amen.

PLEASING GOD OR PLEASING OTHERS

Day
5

Each day, I am called to make a choice, O Lord. I can either be a God pleaser or a people pleaser, but I can't do both. Help me this day to choose wisely and well. Amen.

Yesterday, we learned a powerful lesson about Ananias and Sapphira. Recap in your own words what you learned from that lesson.

_____

_____

_____

_____

Throughout the pages of Scripture, we see a theme that is best summed up by the words spoken by Peter and John in Acts 4:19-20. What do these verses say?

_____

_____

_____

Unfortunately, all too often we make the choice to do what is pleasing to the crowd—or another individual—rather than what we know to be right in God's eyes. In an earlier lesson in our *Daily Victory, Daily Joy* study, we read about the disastrous results of King Herod's people pleasing. Reread Matthew 14:1-11 to refresh your memory of this story. Who were the different people Herod was trying to please? What were the results of his people-pleasing behavior?

_____

_____

_____

It's easy to look at Herod's example and say, "Yes, but he was a wicked king." So let's look at another example about some religious leaders. Turn in your Bible to Matthew 21:23-27. Who was it that came to Jesus asking questions?

_____

_____

_____

The chief priests and religious leaders were afraid to answer Jesus truthfully for two reasons. What are the reasons given in Matthew 21:25-26?

_____

_____

_____

Have there been times when you were afraid to talk about your faith in God because you feared the reaction of others? Explain your answer.

_____

_____

_____

When we think of the stronghold we call "people pleasing," we often forget to include one person in the list of those we aim to please rather than pleasing God. Mark 10:17-22 gives us a great example of who that person is. Who was this man invested in pleasing?

_____

_____

_____

The rich young man was more interested in pleasing himself than in pleasing God! Mark tells us "his face fell" when he heard Jesus' words, because he had great wealth. What does Jesus say about this type of behavior in Matthew 6:24?

_____

_____

_____

Are you trying to serve more than one master? Are you invested in pleasing yourself and others above pleasing God? Talk to Jesus about your need to put Him first in all things and ask Him to give you the strength and courage to say no to others so that you can say yes to Him.

O Lord God, how foolish I am when I say I want to please You but spend my time and energy doing what pleases others. Forgive me, heal me and restore me so that I can give You first place in all things. Amen.

REFLECTION AND APPLICATION

Day 6

Gracious and merciful God, thank You for loving me and sending Jesus to die for my sins. Pleasing You is my goal. Help my actions to support my words. Amen.

Our memory verse for Week Seven talks about the importance of pleasing God. As First Place 4 Health participants, pleasing God is both our goal and desire. This week, we have learned about actions and attitudes that please Him—and attitudes and actions that don't. While doing this study, you have made many choices. Some of these were probably intentional and well thought out, while others were most likely impulsive.

Take a look at the Live It Tracker you have filled out for this week. The Live It Tracker is an excellent tool to help you evaluate your actions when it comes to giving credence to your words that Christ has first place in your everyday life.

Review the entries you have made and then make a list of 10 things you have done this week that were pleasing to God. Then make a list of 10 things you have done that were not in keeping with God's will for your life. This is not a time to judge yourself harshly or make excuses for why you did or didn't do something. It is simply a time to reflect on the information you have been recording for this purpose.

Choices that Pleased God	Choices that Displeased God

After making your list, thank God for helping you to make the choices that were pleasing to Him and ask for His continued guidance so that you can avoid making choices that are displeasing to Him.

> *Lord, all too often my feet are quick to run toward evil. Forgive me for not always taking the straight and level paths that are pleasing to You. Amen.*

REFLECTION AND APPLICATION

Day 7

> *Lord , You are the God of encouragement, and You are pleased when I encourage others. Help me to be a faithful encourager as I reflect Your light in the lives of those who are struggling and in despair. Amen.*

During our Day Four study, we read about a man called Barnabas. Turn in your Bible to Acts 4:36 and write down what we are told about him in that passage.

_____

_____

_____

_____

_____

Barnabas was an encourager! He encouraged others by his words and deeds. When the apostle Paul needed help, Barnabas came alongside him. As part of the First Place 4 Health program, you are asked to do intentional acts that will strengthen and encourage others and give them hope. Your *First Place 4 Health Member's Guide* has a section on the importance of encouragement. Spend some time reading those pages today.

After you have read about encouragement, it's time to practice it! Think of one person in your group who is currently struggling—either in making healthy choices regarding food and exercise, or with a personal problem that is too heavy for him or her to bear. Pray for that person by name, and then call, write or email him or her during the week. Our God is the God of encouragement, and when we encourage others, we are doing what is pleasing to Him.

> *Wonderful Counselor, You encourage me daily as You bring hope and healing into my life. Help me to be an encourager to others as You use me as Your hands and feet, eyes and ears, heart and smile to the hurting and the lost. Amen.*

Group Prayer Requests

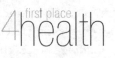

Today's Date: _____

Name	Request

Results

_____

_____

_____

_____

_____

_____

_____

completing the task

SCRIPTURE MEMORY VERSE

However, I consider my life worth nothing to me, if only I may finish the race and complete the task the Lord Jesus has given me— the task of testifying to the gospel of God's grace.

ACTS 20:24

Many of us have a long track record of uncompleted tasks when it comes to personal wellness. We are great starters, but poor finishers. Often, we don't make it to the finish line. Somewhere between the beginning of our journey and reaching of our goals, we become lost, distracted, preoccupied or too discouraged to press on. Paul put it this way: "You were running a good race. Who cut in on you and kept you from obeying the truth?" (Galatians 5:7).

Jesus told a parable that is applicable to this uncompleted-task syndrome that plagues so many of our lives: There once were two brothers. The father came to the first son and asked him to go work in his field. The son said no to his father's request, but later he changed his mind and did as his father asked. When the father asked the second son to work in the field, he immediately said, "I will, sir," but then did not go.

Jesus ended the parable by asking His listeners which of the two sons did what their father wanted. Of course, the answer was the first son who reconsidered his hasty reply and did as his father requested. In telling this parable (found in Matthew 21:28-31), Jesus was telling us that it is not what we say but what we do that matters in the end. Good beginnings without completion are nothing more than good beginnings. Intentional obedience completes the task.

As we begin this week's study, spend a moment or two recalling the times you told God that you would care for your body according to His request but then never completed the task at hand. When you have finished your mental recollection, ask God to help you move forward into victory over these failings as you begin to work through this week's Bible study.

FACING HARDSHIPS

Gracious God, I trust that You are working all things together for Your glory and my good, even when I don't know for sure where I am going or what is happening to me. Help me to put my eternal calling in Christ Jesus before momentary pleasure. Amen.

In order to fully understand what the apostle Paul is teaching us in this week's memory verse, we must first read the verse in context. Our memory verse is part of a farewell address that Paul was giving before setting out on the next leg of his missionary journey. Turn in your Bible to Acts 20:17-24 and read the entire passage, which ends with this week's memory verse.

What specific situation is Paul addressing in this passage?

_____

_____

_____

How had Paul been interacting with the people of Asia during the time he spent serving them?

_____

_____

_____

It appears that serving with great humility had not been easy for Paul. What else do we learn in verse 19?

_____

_____

_____

If you were giving a report of how you interact with your group members, could you, like Paul, say that you were humble and compassionate toward others even when you were being severely tested? Explain your answer.

_____

_____

_____

_____

In Acts 20:20, we learn that Paul did not allow his teaching to be hampered by his opponents. What did Paul continue to do in spite of great opposition?

_____

_____

_____

How is this different from the people-pleasing behavior we learned about in last week's lesson?

_____

_____

_____

Acts 20:20 also tells us that Paul taught publicly and from house to house. How are public worship (such as at a worship service at your church) and small-group participation both part of Christian maturity?

_____

_____

_____

What did Paul tell both Jews and Greeks that they must do?

_____

_____

_____

Why is Paul saying goodbye to the Ephesian elders? Where is he going?

_____

_____

_____

Paul says that he is not certain what will happen to him when he reaches Jerusalem. According to Acts 20:22, why is Paul going there anyway?

_____

_____

_____

In a similar manner, most of us in First Place 4 Health do not know what life will be like when we reach our goals, yet we are compelled by the Spirit to make the journey. Spend the rest of your quiet time praising God that through the power of His Holy Spirit, you are being compelled to press on, even though you cannot always clearly see what lies ahead.

Lord, those who have not heard Your voice and responded to Your call have a hard time understanding what it means to be compelled by Your Spirit. Thank You for giving me the grace to hear Your voice and the courage to follow where You lead. Amen.

Day 2 — HARDSHIPS AND TRIALS

O Lord God, not only do I face an uncertain future, but I also know that I will encounter hardships and trials on the road I am called to travel. Be with me and steady my course. I put my trust in Your unfailing love. Amen.

During yesterday's Bible study, we began looking at the passage of Scripture that contains this week's memory verse. Today, we will pick up where we left off and continue to study Acts 20:17-24. You might want to take a moment to review yesterday's lesson in preparation for today's study. Also reread Acts 20:17-24 and make note of any information the Spirit brings to your awareness that you did not see yesterday.

Why is it important that we take the time to learn what was happening when these words were written?

_____

_____

_____

_____

At the conclusion of yesterday's lesson, we learned that Paul was going to Jerusalem, even though he didn't know what awaited him there. Why was Paul making the journey?

_____

_____

_____

Although Paul did not know what would happen when he finally got to Jerusalem, he did know what would happen along the way. According to Acts 20:23, what was going to happen to Paul? How did he know about these things?

_____

_____

_____

Just as the Holy Spirit warned Paul about the dangers that he would encounter, the Spirit will also prepare you for what lies ahead if you allow Him to do so. Although you are not likely to go to prison for participating in First Place 4 Health, you are sure to encounter times when the way forward will be hard. What are some of the hardships that you might face as you travel on this road to health and wholeness? (Please give this question careful thought—it could include the loss of friendships, giving up certain activities or facing opposition from family members who feel threatened by your new life in Christ. If there is not enough room to record your answer below, make your list in your journal.)

_____

_____

_____

_____

Our memory verse for this week tells us that Paul had been given a specific task. What was that task?

_____

_____

_____

Although we may not be called to go to foreign lands or to preach and teach like Paul, every Christian has been called to testify to the gospel of God's grace. How is First Place 4 Health part of your testimony to God's grace—and the forgiveness in Jesus Christ that makes it possible for you to become a new creation?

_____

_____

_____

The thought of reaching others for Christ Jesus was so great for Paul that he was willing to give his very life in order to accomplish this calling. Now, when Paul says that he considers his life worth nothing in Acts 20:24, he is not saying that he thinks he is a worthless person. Paul knew that he had great value in the kingdom of God. Rather, Paul is saying that compared to the calling he has in Christ Jesus, his life is worth nothing.

_____

_____

_____

Are you willing, like Paul, to endure hardship, considering your life worth nothing at all, in order to testify to the gospel of God's grace? Why or why not?

_____

_____

_____

> *Merciful Savior, You tell me that if I want to follow You, I must deny myself, take up my cross and follow You. Lord, please give me a compassion for the lost that allows me to undergo hardship so that they can learn about Your grace and love. Amen.*

Day 3 — THROWN OFF COURSE

I love You, O Lord my strength. Help me to cling to You when the storms of life threaten to throw me off course. Amen.

In the introduction to this week's Bible study, we read a question that the apostle Paul asked the Galatian Christians. Look back to the beginning of this week's study, or turn to Galatians 5:4 and write Paul's words.

_____

_____

_____

Paul begins by telling these Christians that they were running a good race. The people in this region were avid fans of the Greek Games, including racing events. Just as Jesus taught in parables that the people of his region could easily understand, Paul used the analogy of a runner because his audience could relate to that terminology. What does this tell you about God's eagerness to have us understand the truth of His Word?

_____

_____

_____

During these Greek Games, runners were not judged only on speed but also on how well they ran the race according to the rules. A runner with the fastest time could be disqualified if he did not exhibit sportsmanlike behavior. How might this truth also apply to the way we run the First Place 4 Health race?

_____

_____

_____

Would it be in good form to run in the First Place 4 Health race but follow a different food plan—such as one that produced faster results but robbed your body of vital nutrition?

_____

_____

_____

_____

Although the Galatian Christians had been running a good race, something had happened to them to throw them off course. A group of men called Judaizers had infiltrated the fledgling church after Paul left and convinced the new Christians that belief in Jesus Christ was not enough—they had to add practices such as being circumcised and keep Jewish religious customs to be saved. This same danger is present for us when we begin First Place 4 Health. How do some people threaten the race that we are running?

_____

_____

_____

_____

Write down a time since you began this session when well-intentioned, but misdirected, people tried to convince you that First Place 4 Health was not sufficient for your particular problem. (Remember that one of those people may have been you!)

_____

_____

_____

_____

In Galatians 5:4, what does the apostle Paul say these people have done?

_____

_____

_____

Conclude today's session by thinking about what you are currently doing as part of your First Place 4 Health program. Have you added to the wisdom of keeping Christ first in all things or added other man-made rules to the program? (If you need to review the First Place 4 Health basics, use the information contained in your Member's Kit. Your group leader can help you sort through the material if you are not certain where you have gone astray.)

Sovereign Lord, it is so easy for me to listen to the voice of well-intentioned people instead of simply listening to Your voice and obeying Your commands. Forgive me, Lord, for adding anything that distracts from the gospel of Your grace. Amen.

Day 4 — CHRIST ONLY

Only You, Lord Jesus, can take away my sins. Without You, I am lost. You and You alone can save me. Thank You! Amen.

Yesterday, we learned about a problem in the Galatian churches that was threatening to keep them from running the good race. What was that problem?

_____

_____

_____

How did we apply that truth to our participation in First Place 4 Health?

_____

_____

_____

There is another danger that is even more disastrous than allowing others to convince us that Christ is not enough: the belief that we can save ourselves through our good deeds. Yes, following God's commands through participation in First Place 4 Health is pleasing to Him, but being part of a First Place 4 Health group cannot save us from our sins. Jesus and Jesus alone saves! Paul addressed this problem when he wrote to the Christians in Ephesus. Turn now to Ephesians 2 and read verses 1-10. Note that Paul begins this chapter of Ephesians with a profound truth. Write Ephesians 2:1 in the space below.

_____

_____

_____

In Ephesians 2:2-3, Paul elaborates on his opening statement. Paraphrase what Paul is saying in those verses in your own voice.

_____

_____

_____

According to Ephesians 2:3, were any excluded from the sinful condition that made them objects of wrath? Why or why not?

_____

_____

_____

Were that the end of the story, we would all be doomed! But something happened to save us from our life of disobedience. According to Ephesians 2:4, why did God save us?

_____

_____

_____

Read Ephesians 2:4-5 once, and then read it again, allowing it to sink into the depths of your being. It is by grace we have been saved because of His great love for us! What else do we learn about God in Ephesians 2:4?

_____

_____

_____

Not only does God love us, but He is also rich in mercy! What does the term "rich" in this sentence say to you?

_____

_____

_____

Elsewhere, Scripture describes this rich mercy as God's lavish love—love without limit or condition. Spend some time praising God for His great love and abundant mercy. Let this truth radiate through your entire being. God's love is great and His mercy is rich! What a blessing we have in Christ Jesus our Lord!

Because of His great love and rich mercy, what does Ephesians 2:5 tell us God did for us—and when did He do it?

_____

_____

_____

When we were dead in our transgressions, was there anything we could have done to save ourselves?

> No! We were completely powerless to help ourselves. It is by _____ we
> have been _____ (Ephesians 2:5).

Read Ephesians 2:6-7 and describe what happened next. Why did God choose to lavish His grace on sinners?

_____

_____

_____

Lest there be any doubt in our mind about the sufficiency of Christ after that statement, Paul repeats himself, this time more emphatically. Write Paul's words, as found in Ephesians 2:8, in the space below.

_____

_____

_____

Paul also makes sure we know where salvation *doesn't* come from. What truth does Paul impart in Ephesians 2:9?

_____

_____

_____

Does that leave any room for boasting? Why or why not?

_____

_____

_____

Ephesians 2:10 has a great First Place 4 Health application. Read those words now. Who created us? Who are we created in? And why did God re-create us as new creatures in Christ Jesus? Write your answer as if you were trying to explain this wonder we call grace to someone who does not know Christ.

_____

_____

_____

_____

We are not saved by good works but by grace so that we can do the good works we were created to do! Amazing grace!!

Mighty Savior, the truth of Your grace is more than my finite mind can comprehend. When I was still a sinner, You died for me! How can I ever thank You for Your great love and rich mercy? Amen.

GRACE DEMANDS A RESPONSE

Lord, I am so thankful You chose to shower me with the gift of salvation in Christ Jesus. Help me to show Your grace and love to others in need of Your touch. Amen.

This week, we have been studying the wonders of God's marvelous grace, as found only in Christ Jesus our Lord. However, grace always demands a response on our part. As we learned in yesterday's lesson, we have been saved by grace so that we can do the good works we were created to do! So, while participation in First Place 4 Health (or any other human institution) cannot save us, it can certainly prepare us to respond to the grace we have been given.

Our memory verse for this week tells us how the apostle Paul responded to God's grace. Write that verse, from memory, in the space below.

_____

_____

_____

_____

In order to fully understand Paul's compulsion to preach the gospel, we have to understand the grace extended to Paul by the Lord that Paul now feels compelled to serve. Turn in your Bible to Acts 9 and read verses 1-18, which is the passage that tells us about Paul's miraculous conversion. From other Scripture passages, we know that Paul was a well-educated Pharisee from the prestigious tribe of Benjamin. If anyone could have been saved by keeping the law, it would have been Paul. However, after his conversion, Paul called all those worldly accomplishments "rubbish" when compared to the joy of knowing Jesus Christ as his Lord and Savior.

What accomplishment might you need to leave behind in order to do the good works God created you in Christ Jesus to do? (As you answer this question, remember that one of the things God has called you to do is care for His temple, your body.)

_____

_____

_____

When Jesus appeared to Paul on the Damascus road, He asked Paul (who was then called Saul) a pertinent question. Refer to Acts 9:4 and write the question that Jesus asked Paul.

_____

_____

_____

In last week's study, we learned that what we do to God's people we also do to Him! Using that information, what are you doing when you abuse your body with excess food and insufficient exercise? Explain your answer.

_____

_____

_____

_____

Paul confirms this truth in 1 Corinthians 3:16 and 6:19-20. What does Paul say in those two verses?

_____

_____

_____

In 1 Corinthians 6:20, Paul tells us that we were bought at a price. What was the price God paid for you? (John 3:16 has the answer if you are in doubt.)

_____

_____

_____

Spend the rest of your quiet time today asking God how He wants you to respond to the lavish grace that He has extended to you in Jesus Christ. Use your prayer journal to record your questions and God's answers.

> *Forgive me, Lord, for those times I have abused my body, thinking I was only hurting myself. I know now that when I hurt me, You hurt, too. Thank You for saving me from a life of sin and death. Amen.*

Day
6

REFLECTION AND APPLICATION

Lord, when I was lost, You saved me. When I stood condemned, You redeemed me.
When my life was in shambles, You re-created me. Thank You for Your mercy. Amen.

This week, we learned some powerful truths about the gospel of God's grace
and our responsibility as saved sinners to preach the gospel so that others can
also experience God's love. Today is a day to write your own salvation story.
Begin, as Paul did in writing to the Ephesians, by describing what your life was
like before God saved you. Paul says we were "dead in our transgressions," so
don't be afraid to tell it like it was!

_____

_____

_____

_____

_____

_____

_____

_____

Next, describe what happened—how you first encountered Jesus, as Paul did on
the Damascus road. When did you first become aware that Jesus was calling
you to be one of His disciples?

_____

_____

_____

_____

_____

_____

_____

_____

Finally, talk about your life now that you are a recipient of God's great love and unfathomable mercy. Be sure to include how First Place 4 Health has been part of God's grace in your life. This will become the foundation of your First Place 4 Health testimony.

_____

_____

_____

_____

_____

_____

_____

If you are having trouble with this exercise, take an honest look at whether you are still trying to save yourself instead of solely relying on Christ. It might be a good idea to talk to your group leader, your pastor, or a mature Christian friend.

Gracious God, You invite me to become part of Your family. You extend Your grace to me. You forgive my sins. Help me to always remember that I am saved by Your grace and Your grace alone. Amen.

REFLECTION AND APPLICATION

Day
7

My Lord and my God, I have hidden Your Word in my heart. Help me to use Your Word to proclaim the gospel of Your grace. Amen.

In order to proclaim the gospel of God's grace, it is important that we have God's Word hidden in our heart. The Holy Spirit can, and will, bring those who need to hear what God has done for us into our path when we least expect to encounter them. Memorizing Scripture is part of testifying to the gospel of God's grace!

For the past seven weeks, you have been asked to memorize certain Scripture verses. Today, on this day of reflection and application, you are going to write all seven of those verses from memory in the chart below. Next to each verse, write one way that you have been able to apply the truth found in that verse to your First Place 4 Health program. If you have been diligent in your memorization of God's Word, you will be able to complete this task with ease!

Week	Memory Verse	First Place 4 Health Application
Two		
Three		
Four		
Five		
Six		
Seven		
Eight		

Sovereign and mighty God, You have done such wonderful things for me, and my heart is filled with joy. Help me to share the joy that I have found in You with others who are still living without help and without hope. Amen.

Group Prayer Requests

4 first place
health

Today's Date: _____

Name	Request

Results

_____

_____

_____

_____

_____

_____

our power supply

SCRIPTURE MEMORY VERSE

"Not by might nor by power, but by my Spirit,"
says the Lord Almighty.

ZECHARIAH 4:6

Living within all those who confess Jesus Christ as Lord and Savior is a source of unlimited power—dynamic power! Through the indwelling presence of the Holy Spirit, we can do all things that God asks us to do—even things that from a worldly perspective are impossible.

"With man it is impossible, but with God all things are possible," Jesus declared when His disciples asked Him who could be saved (Matthew 19:26). Those same words were said by the angel Gabriel when he appeared to a young peasant girl to tell her she would soon be the mother of the promised Messiah (see Luke 1:37). Paul would tell the young (and perhaps timid) Timothy that God did not give us a spirit of timidity but a Spirit of power, of love and of self-discipline (see 2 Timothy 1:7). Elsewhere in Scripture, we are told that the same mighty power that raised Jesus Christ from the grave lives in all who believe that Jesus died for their sins and rose from the dead.

However, in stark contrast to these words we read about God's power in us, we see Christians living defeated and powerless lives. For them, all things seem impossible, even the little chores that make up their everyday lives. As Jesus said as He healed the woman who had been bent over for 18 years, they are crippled by a spirit; Satan has kept them bound (see Luke 13:11,16). Some of these afflicted souls, like the woman Jesus healed in the synagogue that day, have been part of the Body of Christ for many years. They confess the name of Jesus, but they are not able to experience the freedom that is theirs in Christ Jesus. Jesus promised that when the Son sets us free, we will be free indeed (see John 8:36), but these people are anything but free.

Perhaps in your own life the burden of carrying extra weight for many years, coupled with the affliction caused by not taking proper care of yourself, has left you feeling defeated and bound. You have read self-help books and attended seminars and workshops, but still you are not experiencing the freedom Jesus came to give His people. These books and seminars tell you how to break free, but they don't give you the power to break free. In the end, all they do is increase your sense of failure! But in the midst of our infirmity, at those times when we are in darkness, when we are feeling helpless and hopeless, we hear our God declare, "Not by might nor by power, but by my Spirit, for with man it is impossible, but with God, all things are possible!"

REMAIN FAITHFUL   Day 1

Gracious God, without You I can do no good thing. Yet in and through You, I can do all things according to Your will for me. Keep me close to You this day and always. Amen.

Zechariah was one of God's prophets; a man called to bring God's word to God's people. History tells us that Zechariah's prophecies began two months after Haggai's first message—a message that urged God's people to quit ignoring the shabby condition of God's house and begin to rebuild the Temple, as He desired. God sent Zechariah to encourage and strengthen the people who had just begun rebuilding the Lord's house in obedience to God's word through Haggai.

Our gracious God wanted His people to remain faithful and establish a close relationship with their Lord rather than merely working on a remodeling project. God wanted to use the rebuilding of the Temple as an opportunity to rebuild the faith and trust of the people who had ignored the Lord's voice for way too long. God knew that the physical condition of the Temple was indicative of a much deeper problem.

In the same way, the Lord calls us to enter into a close relationship with Him, even as we restore the body that years of not taking care of ourselves has torn down. Just as God used the prophet Zechariah to remind His people that they needed Him, He uses programs such as First Place 4 Health to remind us that a love relationship with Him is our first priority. In First Place 4 Health, we call this "keeping Christ first in all things."

Zechariah was sent to call God's people into a love relationship with their Lord. How is First Place 4 Health calling you into a love relationship with God, even while you are still in the rebuilding process? List at least three concrete ways that God is using First Place 4 Health to deepen your relationship with Him.

1. _____

2. _____

3. _____

Earlier in today's lesson, we learned that Zechariah was sent to encourage God's people to remain faithful because this rebuilding project was extensive and would take considerable time. How is God using First Place 4 Health to encourage you to remain faithful during the months—and perhaps even years—that you will be in restoration mode? Once again, list three concrete ways you have been encouraged to remain faithful.

1. _____

2. _____

3. _____

Not only was Zechariah called to encourage God's people, but his words were also intended to impart strength. How is our memory verse for this week a source of strength to you as you move forward? Again, list three concrete examples of the ways that God is strengthening you by the power of His Spirit.

1. _____

2. _____

3. _____

Conclude your lesson today by writing a prayer of thanksgiving below or in your prayer journal to the God who sends His Word and His Spirit so that you can accomplish the task He has set before you.

_____

_____

_____

O Lord God Almighty, through the truth of Your Word and the power of Your Spirit, You give me everything I need to do the work You call me to do in First Place 4 Health. How grateful I am that You are my Lord. Amen.

GETTING TO KNOW THE SPIRIT

Spirit of love and power, help me to know You in new and exciting ways as I complete this study. Amen.

One of the ways that God calls us into a love relationship with Him is by revealing Himself in the pages of His Word. It is by knowing God that we learn to love Him and by loving God that we can truly serve Him. God wants us to know Him on an intimate level. Most Christians who are serious about their faith journey know quite a bit about God, the Father, and Jesus Christ, the Son. But when it comes to knowledge of the work and ministry of the Holy Spirit, most are found wanting. It is easy to understand why the third person of the Trinity used to be called the Holy Ghost!

Much of the confusion about the work and ministry of the Holy Spirit comes from a misunderstanding of the difference between Old Testament teaching and New Testament theology with regard to the Spirit's presence in people's lives. Jesus talked about the importance of understanding the difference between what is taught in the Old and New Testaments in Matthew 13:52. Look up that verse and restate Jesus' words.

_____

_____

_____

_____

Like a wise merchant, we are to draw from the treasures of both the old and the new covenants, but we are not to confuse the two. In writing to Timothy, the apostle Paul stressed the importance of correctly handling Scripture. Read Paul's words in 2 Timothy 2:15. What did Paul urge Timothy to do?

_____

_____

_____

_____

How are you learning to draw out of both the old treasure chest and the new so that you can correctly handle the word of truth?

_____

_____

_____

Have you been faithful to read longer passages of Scripture in addition to completing your daily Bible study? If not, why not?

_____

_____

_____

If you are unsure of how to best read Scripture so that you are exposed to the whole truth of God's Word, use the First Place 4 Health Scripture reading guide found in your Member's Guide. This guide will expose you to both Old and New Testament readings every day. It will give you a firm foundation based on the prophets and the apostles—those called to speak the very words of God!

Turn to 2 Timothy 3:16. In this passage, Paul tells Timothy that all Scripture is God-breathed. Why did Paul used the word "all" to begin this teaching?

_____

_____

_____

Does "all" exclude any part of Scripture? Explain your answer.

_____

_____

_____

Scripture is "God-breathed," or inspired by the Holy Spirit. Since the beginning, the Holy Spirit has brought life and form as God spoke and all of creation came into being. How is the Holy Spirit described in Genesis 1:1-2?

_____

_____

_____

What areas of your life do you need for the Holy Spirit to hover over today, bringing light to your darkness and clarity to your confusion?

_____

_____

_____

_____

The Spirit comes with power. Be still and know that God—God the Father, God the Son and God the Holy Spirit—is actively working in your life, even as you sit in stillness and pray!

> *Father, You have promised to give me wisdom when I need an extra measure of understanding. Please help me to better understand how the Spirit of the living Lord is active in my life today. Amen.*

THE POWER TO RE-CREATE AND RESTORE

Day 3

> *Loving Creator, You have made me and have remade me; given me life and new life. Even now, by the power of the Holy Spirit working within me, You are reforming me into the image of Your Son. Thank You for Your presence in my life. Amen.*

Yesterday, we said that the Spirit of God has been present since the beginning. What was the Spirit's role in creation as described in Genesis 1:1-2?

_____

_____

_____

Although the Spirit has been present since the beginning, the life, death and resurrection of Jesus Christ made the Spirit's power available to all believers. In the Old Testament, the Spirit was God's agent in creation and re-creation, but rather than being an abiding presence, the Spirit was given selectively according to God's purposes. God gave and took away His Spirit according to His eternal plan and purpose.

Read an example of God sending the Spirit to re-create and restore in Ezekiel 37:1-14. You may recognize this passage from the familiar song about the "dry bones." After reading this passage, how is God's Holy Spirit making your dry bones come to life through First Place 4 Health?

_____

_____

_____

_____

We know that God's Spirit was given to Saul when he was anointed king of Israel but taken away when he continued to blatantly disobey the God who had anointed him king. In Psalm 51:11, David offers up a prayer that reflects this truth. What does David pray for in this verse?

_____

_____

_____

_____

Verses like this cause many Christians who have not yet learned to distinguish between Old and New Testament teaching to fear losing their salvation. They do not realize that when Jesus gave His followers the gift of the Holy Spirit, the Spirit would be their inheritance forever! Read this wonderful truth in Ephesians 1:11-14 and spend time praising God for His glory. Record your words below or in your prayer journal.

_____

_____

_____

_____

In Old Testament times, the Spirit was directly connected with the prophets who spoke God's Word. Even as the Bible is God-breathed, every part of a prophet's call and message were the work of the Holy Spirit. Sometimes, the prophets spoke a message of comfort and of promise, while at other times, they spoke a message of warning and rebuke. However, regardless of the content of the message, the prophets always delivered a message that God's people neglected—to their detriment.

In Zechariah 7:12, we learn the fate of those who refuse to hear the words that the Lord sent by His Spirit. What does Zechariah say the people did? What was God's reaction?

_____

_____

_____

Today, God also wants us to pay attention to the truth of His Word—not because He wants to punish us, but because He loves us and wants to bless us! How is First Place 4 Health teaching you to listen to the words the Lord speaks to you through the voice of His Spirit?

_____

_____

_____

In John 16:12-15, Jesus told the disciples an important truth about the Spirit's message. Read this passage in your Bible and write down what you discovered about the Spirit's message.

_____

_____

_____

_____

As Paul tells us in 2 Corinthians 10:5, we must take captive—and demolish—those inner voices that are contrary to the Word of God. Many people lack the Spirit's power in their Christian walk because they are listening to the voices in their head and confusing them with the voice of God's Holy Spirit! One way we learn to recognize the Spirit's voice is to know God's Word! The voice of the Spirit will never contradict what is written in the pages of Scripture.

Read what we are told about testing spirits in 1 John 4:1. How is First Place 4 Health helping you test the spirits and recognize what is really of God?

_____

_____

_____

Conclude today's session by thanking God for sending His Spirit to guide you into all truth.

> *Lord, it is so easy for me to become confused and lose my way. Thank You for sending Your Holy Spirit to remind me of Your words. Thank You for helping me to discern what words are truly from You. Amen.*

Day 4 RESURRECTION POWER

Spirit of the Living Lord, help me to experience the same power that raised Jesus from the dead as I go about my life this day—and always. Amen.

In the opening pages of the New Testament, we read of an event that forever changed the course of human history. The angel Gabriel made two unexpected visits: one to an elderly childless couple, signifying the end of the old covenant; and then, six months later, to a young virgin, signifying the beginning of something new. Turn in your Bible to Luke 1:26-38. This is a very familiar story to most of us, so please read it carefully and listen for God's present-day Word in this passage.

What was the Spirit's role in the birth of Jesus Christ, the long-expected Messiah?

_____

_____

_____

How is the Spirit's work in Luke 1:35 like the Spirit's work in Genesis 1:1-2?

_____

_____

_____

How does the Spirit play that same role when He takes the Word of God and applies it to those areas in us that need new life? Explain your answer.

_____

_____

_____

_____

Just as the Spirit was present at Jesus' physical conception, the Spirit was present at another beginning—the beginning of Jesus' earthly ministry. Read Matthew 3:13-14. What is happening in this passage, and what role does the Holy Spirit play in these events?

_____

_____

_____

After three years of public ministry, the new covenant, sealed with Jesus' blood for the forgiveness of our sins, was ushered in as our Savior was crucified, died and then rose again, conquering death and the power of evil. With the death and resurrection of Jesus Christ, the Spirit's power became accessible to all believers at all times. What did Jesus tell His disciples about His imminent return to the Father in John 16:7?

_____

_____

_____

It was hard for the disciples to grasp what Jesus was saying. But Jesus was telling them that there would be a new Counselor—a Spirit of Truth who would guide them into all truth. Read what Jesus told His grieving disciples about the Holy Spirit in John 16:8-10. Three present-day ministries of the Holy Spirit are listed in this passage. What are they?

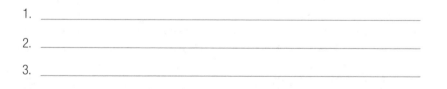

1. _____

2. _____

3. _____

We can see these three vital roles of the Holy Spirit working in and through the First Place 4 Health program. How is the Spirit of God working through First Place 4 Health to convict you of sin (see John 16:8)?

_____

_____

_____

How is the Spirit of God working through the First Place 4 Health program to convince you of the righteousness of Jesus Christ and the forgiveness of sin that is yours today?

_____

_____

_____

_____

How is the Spirit of God working in your life to convince you of the certainty of a future judgment, the necessity of being right before God, and the importance in trusting in Jesus as the One who paid the price for your redemption?

_____

_____

_____

_____

These are not events that come through human effort—they are miracles being brought forth in our lives by the working of the Holy Spirit within us. What does our memory verse for Week Nine tell us about our salvation?

_____

_____

_____

Lord God, how foolish I am when I try to earn what You so freely give. Thank You that the Holy Spirit is within me to convict me of sin so that I can turn to You in repentance and trust in Jesus Christ—and Jesus Christ only—to save me from my sins. Amen.

Day 5 — POWER FROM ON HIGH

O Lord God, thank You for sending the Holy Spirit to be with me forever. Help me to understand His might and power so that I can do the work He equips and empowers me to do. Amen.

After Jesus' resurrection, He appeared to His disciples before ascending into heaven to sit at the right hand of the Father. Just before His ascension, Jesus gave His disciples one last set of instructions. Read those words in Acts 1:3-5.

What did Jesus tell His disciples to do?

_____

_____

_____

Some days later, there was another new beginning—and once again the Spirit of the living Lord was present and active in this event. While the disciples were gathered in the Upper Room, the promised Holy Spirit came in a miraculous display of power! Turn in your Bible to Acts 2:1-12. As you read this passage, imagine that you are one of the disciples assembled in this room as the events take place. What did you experience during this reading? Could you feel the Spirit's presence in the room that day? Why, or why not?

_____

_____

_____

_____

Ordinary men and women, just like us, had received power from on high! Through the power of the Spirit, they were given words to say before rulers and the strength to endure persecution for the sake of the kingdom of God. Truly, this was not about might or power, but about God's Spirit bringing about marvelous things.

Ephesians 1:18-20 gives us information about the Holy Spirit that is the key to living a life pleasing to God. What is Paul's prayer for believers in Ephesians 1:18?

_____

_____

In Ephesians 1:19-20, what does Paul tell us is working in those who believe?

_____

_____

_____

The same dynamic power that raised Jesus from the dead resides in all who believe Jesus died to save them from their sins—and then rose again on the third day to conquer sin and the power of evil. Romans 10:9-10 tells us what gives us access to that power. Read those words and then reaffirm that message!

Another important function of the Holy Spirit is found in Romans 8:16. What is this vital ministry of the Holy Spirit?

_____

_____

_____

_____

If you struggle with assurance of your salvation in Jesus Christ, it is the Spirit who will give you assurance that you are indeed a child of God! Romans 8:26-27 tells us another important fact about the Spirit's ministry. What is the truth found in this passage?

_____

_____

_____

_____

Are you beginning to comprehend why each of us must have the power of the Spirit in our lives if we are going to be able to live a life pleasing to God? Explain your answer!

_____

_____

_____

_____

Conclude by praising God for sending His Holy Spirit to be with you forever!

Lord God, I stand in awe at how You used uneducated men and women to expand Your church here on earth. Truly it was not by might or power, for they had none. All that was done was done by the power of Your Holy Spirit. Amen.

REFLECTION AND APPLICATION

O Lord, through the power living in me, I can live a life that glorifies You.
Without You, I can do no good thing. Amen.

This week, we have learned many new and exciting things about the work of the Holy Spirit. Some of this information may have been new to you. If so, it will take time and repetition for this material to filter into the depths of your being. Remember, one of the functions of the Holy Spirit is to remind you of Jesus' words and guide you into all truth. This is a process that occurs over time. However, even if you do not yet have a complete understanding, it is important that you begin to apply the truths you have learned to your life.

What is one truth from this week's lessons that you can make part of your First Place 4 Health program today?

_____

_____

_____

_____

When Jesus was here on earth, He often asked those who came to Him for help, "What do you want Me to do for you?" Jesus, by the power of the Holy Spirit, is asking that question of you right now! How do you need the Holy Spirit to minister to you today? Write your specific request without explanation or excuse, and then allow the Holy Spirit to take that request and offer it up to God in ways you can't comprehend.

_____

_____

_____

_____

_____

Finally, identify one thing that you are still trying to do in your own might and power instead of relying on the Spirit's power to flow into the weak places of your life. Ask the Spirit to convict you of that sin so that you can surrender to the power of God that is active and working in your life.

_____

_____

_____

Father, You have shown me how the Holy Spirit's presence heralds a new beginning. By His power, help me to begin again today as one forgiven and redeemed by the life, death and resurrection of Your Son, Jesus. Amen.

Day 7

REFLECTION AND APPLICATION

Mighty and powerful God, through the power of Your Spirit, You bring forth all living things. Thank You for calling me to new life in Christ Jesus my Lord. Amen.

As you saw from this study, in the beginning the Spirit of the Lord played an important role in creation. Recall from this week's study what the Spirit was doing when the world was made.

_____

_____

_____

Even now, the Spirit hovers over our darkness and confusion, bringing forth form, clarity, order and definition. Today, sit in silence and let the Holy Spirit hover over you. As He does, allow Him to search you and know you. Allow Him to find those places that are in need of healing and restoration. Allow Him to bring Scripture verses to mind that remind you of God's promises. Today is not about might or power. It is about letting the Spirit of the living Lord do His all-important work in your life.

If you can sit in silence for 20 minutes, please do so. If not, be still for as long as you can. Repeating a Scripture verse will help you stay focused and attentive. This is not about mindlessness—it is about making the purposeful decision to let the Holy Spirit minister to you in your time of need. Conclude your quiet time with a prayer of thanksgiving for the work of the Holy Spirit in your life. You might even want to sing a song about the Spirit's presence in your life.

Spirit of the living God, fall afresh on me as I sit in silence before You. Come beside me and impart strength to my weakness, comfort to my sorrow, peace to my anxious heart and an assurance of God's presence and love in my life. Amen!

Group Prayer Requests

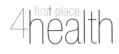

Today's Date: _____

Name	Request

Results

_____

_____

_____

_____

_____

_____

_____

Jesus paid it all

SCRIPTURE MEMORY VERSE
*Therefore, there is now no condemnation
for those who are in Christ Jesus.*
ROMANS 8:1

As we begin to travel down the path that leads to health, wholeness and living a lifestyle that is pleasing to God, one thing quickly becomes evident: We can't move forward and look back at the same time. Getting past a less-than-perfect past is a challenge we all face. Failures, regrets, mistakes, sins, guilt and shame are a heavy burden for our weary shoulders to bear.

To make matters worse, until we get rid of those negative thoughts and emotions, we probably won't be able to get rid of the pounds and inches, either. We will not be able to stop using food to deal with our emotions until we have dealt with the emotions that have fueled that compulsive eating. In a self-perpetuating cycle, our guilt and shame fuels our out-of-control eating, and our out-of-control eating fuels our guilt and shame.

In Romans 7:21-24, Paul wrote the following:

> So I find this law at work: When I want to do good, evil is right there with me. For in my inner being I delight in God's law; but I see another law at work in the members of my body, waging war against the law of my mind and making me a prisoner of the law of sin at work within my members. What a wretched man I am! Who will rescue me from this body of death?

Most of us in First Place 4 Health can echo Paul's words! Like Paul, we have the desire to do what is good, but cannot carry it out (see Romans 8:29). Guilt, shame, mistakes, regrets, failures and sins are part of the universal human condition. But thanks be to God—through Jesus Christ our Lord, there is now no more condemnation!

STRUGGLING WITH SIN

Day
1

Lord God, I am a sinner, saved only by Your grace.
Thank You for redeeming me from a life of sin and death. Amen.

"For all have sinned and fallen short of the glory of God," declared the apostle Paul, a man who knew firsthand the necessity of leaving a painful past behind. As you recall from earlier lessons in this Bible study, Paul had persecuted the Early Church, and in doing so had persecuted the Lord Jesus Christ. Paul even went so far as to describe himself as the worst of sinners, and he used the story of his former way of life to help others realize that in Christ Jesus, their sins could be forgiven, too. Our Week Eight memory verse talked about Paul's desire to preach the gospel of God's grace. As one who had been saved by grace, and grace alone, Paul wanted to share that marvelous grace with others!

"For all have sinned and fallen short of the glory of God." If the story stopped there, we would all stand condemned. But, thanks be to God, there is more! Turn to Romans 3:23-24. What is the rest of God's salvation story?

_____

_____

_____

Drawing on what you have learned in earlier lessons, why does Romans 3:24 say we are "justified freely by his grace"?

_____

_____

_____

Paul preached the gospel of salvation by grace through faith. Once again recalling earlier lessons in this Bible study, what had the false teachers who infiltrated the young churches Paul established tried to do to the gospel of grace that Paul taught?

_____

_____

_____

Paul again emphasized what our life was like before Christ in his letter to Titus, one of his faithful disciples. Turn now to Titus 3:3-5 and summarize what verse 3 says about our former way of life.

_____

_____

_____

During the Day Seven application and reflection time last week, you began to write your salvation story. How does your "what it was like" story compare to what Paul described in Titus 3:3?

_____

_____

_____

_____

But then something happened to change all that! According to Titus 3:4, what was this?

_____

_____

_____

And when God our Savior appeared, what happened (see Titus 3:5)?

_____

_____

_____

Had we done anything to deserve salvation? If not, why did Christ save us?

_____

_____

_____

Merciful Savior, Your grace is too amazing for me to fully comprehend and appreciate! But I know what my life was like before You appeared—and I know that You saved me. I am grateful for Your compassion and love. Amen.

THEN AND NOW

Day 2

When I was still a sinner, You showed Your love for me, O God, by sending Jesus to die for my sins. Thank You for the gift of salvation. Amen.

Our Week Ten memory verse begins with a word that invites us to look at the verses that come before it. Write out this week's memory verse, and then circle the word that invites us to discover why it is there.

_____

_____

_____

In order to understand why Paul is making this bold declaration, we must go back into Romans 7. But before looking at the final verses of Romans 7, underline the word "now" in the memory verse you just wrote out. What does the word "now" imply? Why do you think Paul included it in this sentence?

_____

_____

_____

Perhaps the best way to comprehend why Paul is using the word "now" is to remember what our life was like before Christ. Romans 5:8 repeats a truth that we studied in earlier lessons. What does this verse say?

_____

_____

_____

According to the first part of Romans 6:23, what had our former way of life earned us?

For the _____ of _____ is _____.

Once again, the little word "but" tells us that things have changed. What is the truth contained in the last part of Romans 6:23?

But the _____ of _____ is eternal life in _____ _____ our _____.

What is the difference between wages and a gift?

_____

_____

_____

_____

Our works had earned us death, but God's gift of grace was eternal life. When we were still sinners, we deserved condemnation, but now there is no condemnation for those who are in Christ Jesus! After contemplating that marvelous truth, write a prayer below or in your journal thanking God for giving you the gift of life.

_____

_____

_____

_____

_____

Lord God almighty, even my finest deeds could not save me from my sins. Only Jesus, the Lamb of God, could make me right with You. Thank You for Your incredible gift of salvation. Amen.

Day 3   AT WAR

Thank You, wonderful Savior, for coming to save me from a life of destruction. On my own I can do no good thing, but in and through You, I can become all that You created and called me to be. Amen.

At the beginning of yesterday's lesson, we made note of the word "therefore" in Romans 8:1, our memory verse for this week. Recall from that lesson what the word "therefore" invites us to do.

_____

_____

_____

In order to understand why Romans 8:1 begins with the word "therefore," we must go back to the teaching that precedes the verse. Romans 7:14-25 is a passage to which most of us who struggle to overcome negative behaviors and destructive habits can readily relate. Read this passage and then summarize what Paul is saying in your own voice.

_____

_____

_____

Was there a time this past week when your good intentions and sinful desires were at war with each other? Write out this situation below.

_____

_____

_____

In other passages, Paul describes this battle as one between the new man and the old man—or between the new creation in Christ Jesus and the sinner condemned to death. In Romans 7:24, Paul decries his wretched condition and longs for someone to rescue him from the body of death that wages war against his spirit. And yet, even as Paul speaks these words, he knows that there is One who can save him. What does Paul say about this Person in Romans 7:25?

_____

_____

_____

In your *First Place 4 Health Member's Guide*, there is a description of the Four-Sided Person. What are the four aspects of our being?

1. _____

2. _____

3. _____

4. _____

Even though we talk about these four aspects separately, they are interrelated; what we do in one area impacts the other three. When we live a balanced life, these four parts of our life are equal and in agreement. We are whole and complete and can function with integrity. However, when the four quadrants are disproportionate, we become fragmented. The interrelated aspects of our being vie with one another for power and control. When we are fragmented, either one part dominates or all parts fail.

In Romans 7:14-25, Paul writes that he was at war with himself. The desires of his physical body were at war with the desires of his spirit. How about you? In the table below, write about which parts of your being are in agreement with your physical, mental, emotional and spiritual goals, and which parts are resistant to growth and change. For instance, if your negative thoughts keep you from eating healthy food, your mind (and therefore your emotions) are at war with your body and spirit.

PHYSICAL	MENTAL
EMOTIONAL	SPIRITUAL

What do you need to do to bring balance and harmony to all parts of your being?

_____

_____

_____

_____

O Loving Lord, You are the only one who can save me from this inner turmoil that keeps me in defeat and despair. Please touch my life and make me whole. Amen.

NO CONDEMNATION

Almighty God, in Your great salvation plan, You provided a way for me to obtain eternal life. Thank You for calling me to faith in Jesus Christ my Lord. Amen.

Our memory verse for the week contains both a statement and a qualifier. Write out this week's memory verse, and then draw a circle around the statement and a rectangle around the qualifier.

_____

_____

_____

Why do you think Paul put in this qualifier?

_____

_____

John 3:16-18 can help us understand Paul's words. Turn to those verses now. (If you attended church and Sunday School as a child, John 3:16 is probably one of the first Bible verses you memorized!) According to John 3:16, what prompted God to send His One and only Son to earth in human form?

_____

_____

What does the word "so" in this verse tell us about the extent of God's love?

_____

_____

Although God did the sending and Jesus came to earth in obedience to His Father's will, we have a responsibility, too. What does John 3:16 tell us is our part?

_____

_____

_____

What will happen to those who believe in Jesus?

_____

_____

_____

_____

Although many people think of our God as a God of wrath and condemnation—a cynical sadist just waiting to punish people for the slightest wrongdoing—John 3:17 tells a much different story. According to this verse, what did Jesus come to do—and not do—in accordance with His Father's plan and purpose for humankind?

_____

_____

_____

_____

John 3:18 describes two classes of people. Who are they, and what is their fate?

_____

_____

_____

_____

How do Jesus' words in John 3:18 help you to understand the truth stated in this week's memory verse?

_____

_____

_____

_____

If you are in Christ Jesus, there is no condemnation. Your sins are forgiven. You can go in peace!

O Lord, I often make salvation so complicated. But Your words are simple and straightforward—those who believe in Jesus are heirs of eternal life. Thank You! Amen.

THE VERDICT IS IN

O Lord God, You are my strong defender, the One who upholds my case and
comes to my assistance when I am in distress. You have defeated the enemy,
and because I believe in You, I can also be victorious. Amen.

During yesterday's lesson, we looked at John 3:16-18. Summarize what you learned from your study of those three verses.

_____

_____

_____

The word "condemn" brings up images of a trial. The jury has deliberated the case and the verdict is in. The accused will either be condemned or acquitted. Jesus continues this teaching in John 3:19-21, using the illustration of a verdict being reached. As you read these verses, picture a courtroom scene in your mind. Write about the verdict as though you were covering a trial, being sure to recap the evidence presented to help the jury make their decision.

_____

_____

_____

_____

Once again, there are two classes of people described in this passage. What two types of people do John 3:20-23 describe?

_____

_____

Jesus uses the analogy of light and darkness in these verses. According to John 3:21, who are the ones who come into the light?

_____

_____

_____

Revelation 12:10 tells us about another person who is present at a trial. Who is that person, and what does he do day and night?

_____

_____

_____

While Jesus came to take away our guilt and shame, what does Satan try to do?

_____

_____

_____

We can recognize the difference between the voice of the Holy Spirit convicting us of sin and the voice of Satan accusing us of sin, in that along with the Spirit's conviction, there is always an assurance of pardon through Christ's righteousness on our behalf. Satan's accusations leave no room for redemption or forgiveness. How is First Place 4 Health part of the Spirit's work as He convicts you of sin and then assures you there is no condemnation because you are in Christ Jesus? Be thoughtful and thorough in your answer.

_____

_____

_____

_____

_____

O Lord, Your mercies are new every morning. Thank You for forgiving me and allowing me to begin again through the miracle of new birth in Christ Jesus. Amen.

Day 6 — REFLECTION AND APPLICATION

Gracious God, thank You for the assurance that my sins are forgiven because Jesus bought me at a price. My responsibility is to honor You with my body, because I belong to You. Amen.

Because there is no condemnation for those who are in Christ Jesus, we can always begin again, no matter how miserably we have failed. This week, we have looked at many verses from Romans, the book of the Bible in which we find this week's memory verse. Today, we will contemplate one more passage.

Turn to Romans 8:38-39. Read this passage and then list the things that cannot separate us from the love of God that is in Christ Jesus our Lord.

_____

_____

_____

_____

After compiling your list, spend time thinking about how you have allowed your own guilt and shame to keep you from experiencing God's great love. List some of these below or in your prayer journal.

_____

_____

_____

_____

_____

_____

Nothing can separate us from God's love, but our attitudes can keep us from experiencing God's love. Conclude today's session by contemplating this week's memory verse as it relates to Romans 8:38-39. There is no condemnation! End your reflection and application time with a prayer of thanksgiving to the God who saved you from your sins!

Lord God, help me to grasp the truth that nothing, absolutely nothing, can separate me from Your great love. Forgive me for the times I allow my guilt and shame to interfere with my relationship with You. Through the power of Your Holy Spirit, give me assurance that I am Your beloved child. Amen.

REFLECTION AND APPLICATION

Day 7

Lord Jesus, You died for me. Help me to live for You. Amen.

Because there is no condemnation in Christ Jesus, every day can be a new beginning in First Place 4 Health! Today, we are going to celebrate new beginnings by making a collage of new things that symbolize our new birth in Christ.

Begin by taking a sheet of paper and writing "New Beginnings" across the top. Next, find 12 pictures or symbols that represent new beginnings. It could be babies (human or animal), plants putting forth new growth, a new piece of clothing, or even a haircut. Be imaginative and creative in your design. The important thing is that you find a collection of items that speak to you of new birth, new beginnings and new opportunities. After selecting 12 pictures or symbols, glue them to the paper titled "New Beginnings." You will be sharing your creation with your First Place 4 Health group this week, so take some time to write down below what each item in your collage means to you.

_____

_____

_____

_____

_____

_____

_____

_____

Thank You, Creator God, for allowing me to reflect Your image and likeness when I create things that glorify You. Amen.

Group Prayer Requests

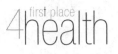

Today's Date: _____

Name	Request

Results

_____
_____
_____
_____
_____
_____
_____

trust in the Lord

SCRIPTURE MEMORY VERSE
Those who know your name will trust in you,
for you, Lord, have never forsaken those who seek you.
PSALM 9:10

"Blessed is the one who has believed that everything the Lord has said will be accomplished," exclaimed Elizabeth (see Luke 1:45). "The Lord is faithful to all his promises and loving toward all he has made," David echoed in Psalm 145:13. In those sage words is found the secret to daily victory and daily joy. For until we believe in the depths of our heart that our God is faithful—that He will fulfill all His promises to us—we will not be able to apply what we have learned to our everyday lives. Our learning will merely be information that does not lead to transformation. "Trust" is what the Bible calls that deep-seated belief that God will do everything exactly as He has promised:

- Trust in the truth of God's Word
- Trust that God is faithful
- Trust that God is loving toward us
- Trust that God is working all things together for His glory and our good—even when circumstances tell us otherwise
- Trust that relinquishes the right to say, "But Lord!" or "What if?"

During the course of this study, you have learned many new behaviors. If you have been faithful to the spiritual component of First Place 4 Health, you have grown in grace and knowledge of the Lord Jesus Christ and your relationship with Him has grown deeper. Indeed, there is a greater level of trust than when you began this Bible study. If you have been faithful to the emotional and mental components, your thoughts are clearer and the quality of your relationship with others—and yourself—has improved. Balance and harmony have re-

placed the war waging within. If you have been faithful to the physical component, you have lost pounds and inches (or you've maintained your weight if you
have already reached your goal).

SONGS OF PRAISE

*O Lord Most High, it is right that I sing praise to You with my
whole heart, for You have been good to me. Amen.*

During this study, we have seen the importance of being able to correctly inter-
pret Scripture. In 2 Timothy 2:15, the apostle Paul exhorts us to:

Present ourselves to God as one _____ , a _____ who does
not need to be _____ and who _____ _____
the _____ of _____ .

How has completing this Bible study helped you learn more about correctly
handling the Word of God?

_____

_____

_____

During this study, we have learned the importance of reading verses before
and/or after our memory verses so that as we learn the words, we will also understand the context in which they were written. Why is it important to understand the context in which the verse was written?

_____

_____

_____

Our Week Eleven memory verse comes from King David's psalms of praise.
Turn to Psalm 9 and read the first 10 verses of David's song. In verse 1, David
declares his intent to praise the Lord with all of his heart. What does this mean?
How is wholehearted praise different from just going through the motions?

_____

_____

_____

Praise is not David's only intent in writing this psalm. What else does David declare he will do as he sings praises to the name of the Most High (see v. 2)?

_____

_____

_____

_____

Is it possible to wholeheartedly sing praises to the Most High without being glad or rejoicing? Explain your answer.

_____

_____

_____

_____

Psalm 9:3-8 tells us why David feels compelled to sing God's praise with his whole heart—why he is full of joy and gladness. Read these verses carefully and then use them as a template to write your own song of victory. How has God subdued your foes and upheld your right cause during this session of First Place 4 Health? You can either write your victory psalm below or in your journal.

_____

_____

_____

_____

_____

Psalm 9:9-10 combines to make a strong statement of hope, assurance and trust. Verse 9 tells us that the Lord is a refuge and a stronghold. To whom does God provide refuge, and when is He a stronghold?

_____

_____

_____

_____

How has the Lord been a refuge for you during this session of First Place 4 Health? How has He been your stronghold as you have faced the negative situations that threatened to interfere with your journey to health and wholeness?

_____

_____

_____

_____

Psalm 9:10 (this week's memory verse) tells us why those who know God's name will trust in Him. What is that reason?

_____

_____

_____

_____

Spend time praising God with your whole heart! You are seeking His kingdom and His righteousness, putting Him first in all things, and He has never forsaken you!

> *It is good to praise Your name, O Lord Most High. As I sing Your praises, I am filled with joy and gladness. Because I seek You, I can be confident that You will never forsake me.*

THOSE WHO KNOW YOUR NAME　Day 2

> *O Lord God, I will trust in You. I will take refuge in You. I will call on Your name, confident that You will hear my prayer and will respond. Amen.*

On a human level, we divide people by nationality, race, income level, education, achievement and other man-made categories. But with God, there are only two classes of people. Recall those two categories from last week's Bible study (refer to Day Five of Week Ten if you are unsure of the answer). List those two classes of people below.

1. _____

2. _____

In the context of this week's memory verse, we can also say there are two classes of people: those who know God's name and have a trust relationship with Him, and those who do not and still live in doubt and fear. In human relationships, mutual trust is established slowly over time. So it is with our relationship with God. Trust is built over time.

For those of us who come from a family in which our trust was ruptured at a young age, learning to trust God will be a one-small-step-at-a-time process. Little by little, over time, we must come to know that God is faithful and deserving of our trust. Just reading about God's trustworthiness in the Bible is often not enough to repair the trust that was ruptured in our childhood. We must experience God's faithfulness firsthand before we will be able to trust again.

God, who knows our history, waits patiently for us to come to the place where we can wholeheartedly trust Him. And not only does He wait patiently, but He also gives us abundant evidence of His faithfulness and love in the process. What a wonderful God we serve!

In our modern society, we talk a lot about wanting peace and joy. However, Romans 15:13 shows us that there is a correlation between joy, peace and trust. Turn to that verse and write it out below.

_____

_____

_____

_____

Once you have written out the entire verse, circle the little word "as." "As" in this instance means "in equal measure to." What is thus the correlation between joy, peace and trust?

_____

_____

_____

_____

How do we increase our ability to trust God so that we will have more joy and peace—and be overflowing with hope? By trusting Him! Each time we trust God, He proves Himself faithful and worthy of our trust. Trust begets trust, which in turn builds more trust in a never-ending upward cycle.

How has God proven Himself worthy of your trust this session? Summarize the ways you have trusted Him—and the ways God has proven Himself worthy of that trust.

_____

_____

_____

_____

_____

David was a man who had, over time, learned to trust in God at all times and in all circumstances. Read what he says in Psalm 27:1-3. What were David's circumstances, and what was David's trust?

_____

_____

_____

_____

In a world characterized by instant gratification, genuine trust is a rare commodity. We want immediate results, but, as we have seen, developing trust takes time. Identify one small thing that you can trust God with in the week ahead. Determine to give God an opportunity to prove Himself faithful by committing that one small thing to God in prayer now. Use your prayer journal to record how you will trust God—and then be sure to return to that entry next week and record how God has been faithful!

> _O Lord God, I will be strong, take heart and wait for You, because I know that You have never forsaken those who trust in You. Amen._

THE STRENGTH TO CHOOSE

Day 3

> _Faithful Father, when I am afraid, I will trust in You. When I am anxious, I will cast my cares on You. When I am in need, I will depend on Your goodness. Amen._

Like all other Christian virtues, trust is a choice—a conscious choice to believe that our God is faithful and that His words are true. Left to our own devices, we would be doubtful and skeptical. It is only by the power of God's Holy Spirit that we have the ability to do God's will!

Throughout Scripture, we see God's people using the words "I will" to affirm their decision to do the right thing—even when it goes against their own natural inclinations. Doing what is pleasing to God is not a random and mindless act. Pleasing God is an intentional act of our volition—our will. Saying "I will" indicates that we have weighed the options and made a conscious choice. In First Place 4 Health, we call this intentional act of volition "mindfulness."

"Volition" literally means the power to choose—the strength of will to make our own decisions. In Mark 12:30, Jesus tells us that the most important thing is to "Love the Lord your God with all your heart and with all your soul and with all your mind and with all your strength." In First Place 4 Health, we use that verse as the foundation for the four-sided person, with strength being about the physical component of the First Place 4 Health program. However, in the original language, the word used for "strength" is not about physical prowess. The strength Jesus is referring to is strength of volition, or the power to make the right choice. No matter what we say about our faith in God, until we have the power to choose what is right, all our pious words are exactly that—pious words. In 1 Corinthians 4:20, the apostle Paul puts it this way:

For the _____ of _____ is not a _____ of _____
but of _____ .

Trust is a choice, an act of our volition. It is also a moment-by-moment decision. We either choose to trust in the Lord or choose to give in to doubt and fear. We can trust in God or in things that are sure to fail us, but we can't do both.

One thing that is sure to fail us is our own understanding! Turn to Proverbs 3:5 and write down who it is that we are to trust—and whom we are not to trust.

_____

_____

_____

John 7:17 contains another truth about this thing called trust. Read that verse now and record what you find.

_____

_____

_____

Just as trust is often ruptured in our early childhood, so is volition. Many of us had authority figures impose their will on us instead of empowering us to make right choices. As a result, our power to choose is badly damaged. Our strength to love God as He deserves gives way to people-pleasing. The ability to let our yes be yes and our no be no gives way to doing what others want us to do. Restoration of volition—the power to choose—is an integral part of our path to healing and wholeness. Turn to Romans 12:1-2. What does Paul call this process?

_____

_____

_____

_____

We must learn how to choose to trust in the Lord, and that learning process takes time. It also takes listening to what God teaches us about trusting Him. Turn to Proverbs 3:5. According to that verse, how are we to trust in the Lord?

_____

_____

_____

_____

What else did we learn during our Day One Bible study that we are to do with all our heart?

_____

_____

_____

_____

What happens to our relationship with the Lord when we are not wholehearted in our devotion?

_____

_____

_____

_____

How is being wholehearted in our devotion synonymous with putting Christ first in all things?

_____

_____

_____

In Proverbs 3:6-7, we are told what trusting God with our whole heart looks like when applied to our life. How does trust manifest itself in our daily lives, on a practical level?

_____

_____

_____

_____

What will be the result of trusting in the Lord, acknowledging Him in all our ways and shunning evil, according to Proverbs 3:8?

_____

_____

_____

_____

For those of us in First Place 4 Health, this is an awesome promise! Health for our body and nourishment for our bones is one of our primary goals! Trust breeds trust, and trust is a choice. What will you choose today, and why?

_____

_____

_____

_____

O Lord God, You know that trust is difficult for me. Yet little by little, You are proving Yourself faithful. Help me to trust You more and more so that my peace and joy will increase in proportionate measure. Amen.

AN APPROPRIATE RESPONSE

*Lord God, You ask me to trust You rather than lean on my own understanding.
Today, I will acknowledge You in all my ways—especially the way I care for my
body, because it is the temple of Your Holy Spirit. Amen.*

During our Week Eight, Day Five study, we learned that grace demands a response, and that trust is one of the appropriate responses grace demands. Turn to Romans 8:32 and read about God's ultimate act of faithfulness—and the reason why we can always trust Him.

Paul made his statement into a question. Write Paul's thoughts in your own words so they become a bold statement of faith and trust in the God of grace.

_____

_____

_____

_____

In Romans 8:32, Paul says God will graciously give us all things. How is this similar to Jesus' words in Matthew 6:33, the core verse of First Place 4 Health?

_____

_____

_____

What blessings has God given you during this session of First Place 4 Health as you have sought His kingdom and His righteousness?

_____

_____

_____

_____

Perhaps the greatest challenge for modern-day believers is to trust that Christ will come again in glory to redeem His faithful people from this corrupt world. The first-century Christians expected Jesus to return during their lifetime, but it has now been more than 2,000 years since Christ ascended into heaven—and we are still waiting. The apostle Peter addressed this problem in 2 Peter 3:8-9.

Ask the Spirit to give you a clear mind as you read Peter's words, and then write down the truth that Peter is telling us with regard to God's timing.

_____

_____

_____

In 2 Peter 3:9, Peter talks about God's patience—patience that we often confuse for slowness. Why, according to Peter, is God being patient with regard to Jesus' return to this world?

_____

_____

_____

Think of those you know (perhaps even members of your own family) who do not yet have saving faith in the Lord Jesus. As you think of them, pray for their salvation, and then thank God that He is patiently waiting so that all may come to repentance.

How is First Place 4 Health preparing you for the day that Jesus will return? How are you managing the good things that He has entrusted to your care—especially as it applies to your physical body?

_____

_____

_____

God has given you a wonderfully made body to do His work here on earth. You are called to be His witness, and part of that sacred trust is caring for His sacred temple, your body. If Jesus were to return tonight, would He find you trusting in His name and doing what pleases Him? Why or why not?

_____

_____

_____

Lord, You have given me everything that I need to live a life of godliness. Help me to always remember to care for the things that You have entrusted to me. Amen.

WEAVING IT ALL TOGETHER

Lord God, You teach me the way I should go and surround me with love and compassion. Thank You for being the faithful God in whom I can trust. Amen.

During the Day Six and Seven reflection time, you will be preparing to give your First Place 4 Health testimony and sharing your daily victories and joys with the group. Each week during this study, you have been asked to memorize a Scripture verse that was specifically selected because of its applicability to First Place 4 Health and this Bible study. In the chart below, please write all 10 of these memory verses. Then, next to each verse, write how this verse and that week's lessons have given you daily victory and daily joy in Christ.

Week	Memory Verse	Lesson and Application
Two		
Three		
Four		
Five		
Six		

Week	Memory Verse	Lesson and Application
Seven		
Eight		
Nine		
Ten		
Eleven		

Conclude by thinking about the most important lesson that you learned during this study. Write this in the space below, and then explain why this particularly stuck out in your mind.

_____

_____

_____

_____

Faithful Father, You have promised to complete the good work You have begun in me. Thank You for giving me the perseverance and stamina to complete this study. Amen.

REFLECTION AND APPLICATION

Gracious God, part of my faith journey is sharing my experience, strength and hope with others—and listening to their stories as well. Ultimately, Lord, my story is a story of Your goodness and grace extended to me in Jesus Christ my Lord. Amen.

During the fourth week of *Daily Victory, Daily Joy,* you were asked to envision the progress you would have made by the end of this study. Your vision was not just physical weight loss—it also included positive changes in the other aspects of your being. As we begin the final week of *Daily Victory, Daily Joy,* it is time to go back and see if you have realized these goals and expectations. Refer back to the introduction section of Week Four as you complete the following charts:

Aspect of My Being	My Vision and Goal for this Session
Physical	
Mental	
Emotional	
Spiritual	

Aspect of My Being	What I Have Actually Achieved this Session
Physical	
Mental	
Emotional	
Spiritual	

If you have not realized your goals, you need to ask yourself why. This is not to condemn yourself, but so that you can change the behaviors that kept you from realizing all that you had hoped for during this session of First Place 4 Health. God is always faithful to do His part. Honest assessment of our progress allows us to do our part as well.

Conclude today's reflection and application time by meditating on the victories Christ has given to you. Thank Him for giving you the strength to overcome the challenges in your life and spend some time praising Him for the blessings He has provided to you. Say a special prayer of thanksgiving for the people He has brought into your life who have helped you along the way—and thank Him for the revelations you have learned during this session.

Merciful Savior, You have given me a story unlike anyone else. Yet all those who know Your name have a common element, no matter how diverse the other elements of their story may be. We all know Your name and trust in You as the source of our salvation. You are our eternal hope of glory. Amen.

REFLECTION ID APPLICATION Day 7

The Lord has done great things for us, a we are filled with joy!
Thank You, Lord, that all Y have promised will be
accomplished accordi o Your Word. Amen.

Congratulations! You are almost at the end of this l of your First Place 4 Health journey. Next week, you will celebrate with you oup the daily victory and daily joy that Jesus our Lord has given to you durii this session. You will have an opportunity at this time of celebration to brie share the highlights of your journey with the others in your First Place 4 He h group.

During Week Twelve, rather than a day-to-day Bit study, you will find daily reflection questions that will help you write your stimony for the victory celebration. You have worked on segments of your s. y in prior reflection and application days, so you might want to go back and view those days before you begin writing. You might also want to review tl nemory verses and lessons covered during this study. You do not need to list em all, but be sure to include the major lessons you have learned throughout is 12-week session.

As you begin to prepare for your victory celebration, s time to contemplate your next First Place 4 Health session. Perhaps your up has already selected their next Bible study and has set the beginning date r the next session. If not, be proactive and talk to the others in your group ut your desire to travel on with them in your quest for health, wholeness l living a lifestyle pleasing to God. Be sure to look over the list of Bible st es and help your group select the study that will most closely fit your particular group's needs.

May God bless you as you begin to write down words that will encourage and strengthen others—and add to your personal testimony that gives Jesus Christ first place in your life.

Gracious Lord, I thank You for allowing me to make this First Place 4 Health journey. I now commit my future plans to You, knowing that as I choose to walk in Your will and in Your ways, my plans will succeed. Amen.

Group Prayer Requests

Today's Date: _____

Name	Request

Results

_____

_____

_____

_____

_____

_____

_____

time to celebrate!

To help you shape your brief victory celebration testimony, work through the following questions in your prayer journal:

Day One: List some of the benefits you have gained by allowing the Lord to transform your life through this 12-week First Place 4 Health session. Be sure to list benefits you have received in the physical, mental, emotional and spiritual realms of your being

Day Two: In what ways have you most significantly changed *mentally*? Have you seen a shift in the ways you think about yourself, food, your relationships or God? How has Scripture memory been a part of these shifts?

Day Three: In what ways have you most significantly changed *emotionally*? Have you begun to identify how your feelings influence your relationship to food and exercise? What are you doing to stay aware of your emotions, both positive and negative?

Day Four: In what ways have you most significantly changed *spiritually*? How has your relationship with God deepened? How has drawing closer to Him made a difference in the other three areas of your life?

Day Five: In what ways have you most significantly changed *physically*? Have you met or exceeded your weight/measurement goals? How has your health improved during the past 12 weeks?

Day Six: Was there one person in your First Place 4 Health group who was particularly encouraging to you? How did their kindness make a difference In your First Place 4 Health journey?

Day Seven: Summarize the previous six questions into a one-page testimony, or "faith story," to share at your group's victory celebration.

As you celebrate your daily victory and daily joy in First Place 4 Health, this is our heartfelt prayer for you: *The LORD bless you and keep you; the LORD make his face shine upon you and be gracious to you; the LORD turn His face toward you and give you peace, as you keep Him first in all things* (from Numbers 6:24-26).

Daily Victory, Daily Joy
leader discussion guide

For in-depth information, guidance and helpful tips about leading a successful First Place 4 Health group, spend time studying the *First Place 4 Health Leader's Guide*. In it, you will find valuable answers to most of your questions, as well as personal insights from many First Place 4 Health group leaders.

For the group meetings in this session, be sure to read and consider each week's discussion topics several days before the meeting—some questions and activities require supplies and/or planning to complete. Also, if you are leading a large group, plan to break into smaller groups for discussion and then come together as a large group to share your answers and responses. Make sure to appoint a capable leader for each small group so that discussions stay focused and on track (and be sure each group records their answers!).

week one: welcome to *Daily Victory, Daily Joy*

During this first week, welcome the members to your group, provide a brief overview of the First Place 4 Health program, explain what is expected of the participants at each of the weekly meetings, and collect the Member Surveys. (See the *First Place 4 Health Leader's Guide* for a detailed outline of how to conduct the first week's meeting.)

week two: not beyond our reach

Begin today's lesson by talking about the importance of setting goals as it applies to First Place 4 Health. Remind the group members that unless they plan to succeed, their greatest intentions will fail!

After talking about the importance of setting goals, have someone in the group read Luke 9:51 out loud. Lead a discussion on the word "resolutely" and how that word can help them reach their First Place 4 Health goals.

This week, the members spent a considerable amount of time looking at obstacles that stand between them and success in First Place 4 Health. Ask your group why identifying obstacles before they begin is important.

Considering the cost is an important aspect of goal setting. Discuss how participation in a First Place 4 Health group has a cost in terms of both time commitment and materials. Then talk with your group about the higher cost of carrying excess weight, buying plus-size clothing, and the toll that extra pounds will take on their physical bodies.

Ask the group members to share stories of diet and exercise programs that did not reveal the full "cost" of their program up front.

An excuse is just a lie disguised as a reason. Ask each group member to identify one excuse that he or she has been using for not caring for his or her body as God commands.

It is easy to begin a new diet and exercise program, but it is much harder to sustain that effort over time. Talk about the importance of persevering in the First Place 4 Health program. Ask what would have happened if Jesus had allowed the obstacles and distractions He faced to keep Him from reaching Jerusalem.

The Day Six reflection is about completing the "when I lose weight, then I will . . ." sentence. Ask each person to tell the group about one of his or her answers to this question. Be sure to give everyone—even the shy and new members of your group—an opportunity to talk.

We all have family "obligations" that threaten to sabotage our First Place 4 Health efforts. Once again, ask each group member to share one obligation he or she has to deal with—and the creative solution that he or she will put in place to solve this problem. As before, be sure that everyone is invited and encouraged to share!

Close in prayer, asking for God's blessing as your group begins this session of First Place 4 Health.

week three: words for the wise traveler

The introduction to this week's study began by asking participants to write out their goals and expectations in all four aspects of their being. Ask each person in your group to read their goals out loud so that the group members can hold that person accountable. Be sure each person has time to read his or her goal statement—and don't allow cross-talk in order to keep the shyer members of your group comfortable with this exercise.

The "letting your yes be yes and your no be no" concept will be foreign to some in the group. Most of us are used to talking about what we will do rather than just doing it! So spend time talking about how doing is different from talking.

Lead a discussion about the difference between boasting and being submissive to the Spirit's leading.

The story of Peter's denial of Jesus will probably be familiar to most people in your group. So ask your group members to listen with new ears as you read Luke 22:54-62. Then talk about how Peter's bravado kept him from doing what Jesus asked him to do.

Another example of a boast that produced disastrous results is found in the story of Herod's execution of John the Baptist in Matthew 14:3-9. Ask your group to talk about how people-pleasing can produce disastrous results for them as well.

Our physical, mental, emotional and spiritual goals can often be described as "much dreaming" and "using many words" (from our Day Five study). Put the words "much dreaming," "using many words" and "taking action" on a white-board or flip chart. Ask the group to describe each of these statements. Have someone in the group record each person's answers.

Summarize what this week's lessons taught about the danger of making vows. Once again, have someone record the group's responses.

week four: friends and foes

This week's lessons focus on friends and foes. Before the meeting, ask various members in your group who are comfortable sharing to talk about the people, places and things they have identified as harmful—and as helpful.

Satan is a master of disguise. Talk about the many forms he takes, as outlined in the Day One study.

Write the word "prowl" on your whiteboard or flip chart, and then ask your group to describe what images that word brings to their minds.

Have the group repeat 1 John 4:4 in unison!

The phrase "as a roaring lion" does not mean that Satan is a roaring lion. Talk to your group about why analogies are used in Scripture to help us understand spiritual truth.

We don't have to be prey to Satan's wiles—we can pray. Write "prey" and "pray" on your whiteboard or flip chart, and then talk about how we can pray or become prey.

Ask your group to summarize what they have learned about the devil during this week's lesson. Have a group member record everyone's answers. Encourage members to be honest—and creative—in their answers.

Not all foes are roaring lions. The little foxes described in Day Seven are a very real threat to most of us. Ask your group members to talk about the "little foxes" in their lives.

End today's lesson with a prayer, praising Jesus for overcoming sin and death so that we can have daily victory and daily joy.

week five: our battle hymn

Begin today's session by asking a member of your group to read Paul's words in Ephesians 6:12.

During this week's study, members read about many of the weapons we fight with that are not the weapons of the world. List the three weapons you feel your group needs to learn more about on a whiteboard or flip chart. Lead a discussion about each of these weapons and how they apply to First Place 4 Health.

Many members may be finding it difficult to spend quiet time with God. Talk about the importance of quiet time and how spending time with God each day helps ward off the attacks of the enemy. (Refer to your First Place 4 Health Member's Guide for more information on how to set up a quiet time.)

Praising God is not something that most of us think of as a weapon, but the Bible assures us that it is a powerful defense against the attacks of the enemy. Lead your group in a prayer of praise. If you (or someone in your group) are musically inclined, you could even sing a praise song!

Write down each piece of spiritual armor described in Ephesians 6:13-18 on your whiteboard or flip chart. Ask your group to identify the opposing weapons the world often employs to fight battles. Be sure a member records your group's answers.

Have your group read Hebrews 4:12 out loud, and then lead a discussion about how this verse is part of our daily victory and daily joy in First Place 4 Health.

Ask one of your group members who is a true prayer warrior to talk about how prayer is a strong defense against the enemy.

Put the word "stronghold" on your whiteboard or flip chart, and then talk about the two different types of strongholds we learned about during this week's lesson.

Close with a prayer of praise. Be sure to incorporate God's Word in this prayer so that you will be using three divine weapons at once!

week six: pave the pathway with prayer

At the beginning of the meeting, have your group recite this week's memory verse in unison.

The Lord invites us to call on Him! Write "Call on Me" across the top of your whiteboard or flip chart, and then ask your group to identify times when they are to call on God. Be sure a member records the group's answers.

By now, you should have a good idea where the members of your group are in their level of spiritual maturity. Do you have any members who have not confessed Christ as their Lord? If so, talk about the importance of accepting Jesus into their lives. Invite any person who desires to do so to pray with you!

Psalm 107 is a wonderful passage about how God helps His people when they are in distress. Divide your group into four smaller groups, and then have each group read the portion of Psalm 107 that describes each of the four groups we identified during our Day Two study.

Ask one or two of your group members to share how the Word of God has been part of their healing and restoration.

Write the word "unsearchable" on your whiteboard or flip chart. Ask your group what definitions they discovered when they looked this word up in the dictionary. Have someone record the answers that they provide.

Ask one of your group members to read Acts 12:1-16. This is a wonderful story with many applications, so concentrate your discussion on the answers to prayer that people often overlook.

Conclude by reviewing some of the high points from the first five weeks of this session. Ask your group to share the lessons they feel are most important to their First Place 4 Health success.

week seven: living a life pleasing to God

As you begin this week's lesson, take time to allow each group member to report on the progress he or she has made toward the goals he or she set at the beginning of this session of First Place 4 Health.

Lead your group in a prayer of praise and thanksgiving for the progress that each member has made.

Pleasing God rather than pleasing self or others may be your group members' greatest challenge in First Place 4 Health. During the Day Two study, members were asked to look up seven verses that provided concrete examples of what pleases God. Have someone read each of those seven verses. After each verse, talk about what God is saying pleases Him—and how the members can apply that knowledge to their First Place 4 Health program.

Ask your group to identify the seven detestable things from the Day Three study. Then lead a discussion about "haughty eyes" and "feet that are quick to rush into evil."

Impulsivity is something we need to replace with mindful choices. Put "impulsive" on the board and ask your group to talk about impulsive things they did during the past week that they know were not pleasing to God.

Talk about the importance of integrity from the Day Four lesson. If you have time, read the story of Ananias and Saphira to the group and discuss how their actions are an example of what does not please God.

Barnabas was the son of encouragement and someone whom each of us can learn from. Use this opportunity to talk about the importance of doing intentional acts of encouragement. (The *First Place 4 Health Member's Guide* has a section on encouragement, which you can use as a basis for your teaching.)

week eight: completing the task

It has now been eight weeks since the start of this session of First Place 4 Health. Unfortunately, some of the members of your group may have already gotten off track, so begin the session by asking your members to examine any areas in which they might have started well but are not finishing well. Read Galatians 5:4 and challenge them to get back on track.

Hardship is part of the Christian life, especially when it comes to changing old behavioral patterns and testifying to the gospel of God's grace. Ask your group to talk about hardships they have encountered during this session of First Place 4 Health.

On Day Three, members read about the importance of running in proper form. Guide your group in a discussion about how following only part of First Place 4 Health does not demonstrate running the race in good form.

"Christ only" is a message we must continually proclaim. Most likely, there are some in your group who have confused salvation with rule keeping and who are using First Place 4 Health as a way of earning what God longs to give them. Spend some time talking about the importance of "Christ only."

The lesson of Day Five was that grace demands a response. While First Place 4 Health can't save your members, it can certainly be considered part of a right response to God's grace. Put "grace demands a response" on your whiteboard or flip chart, and then talk about how First Place 4 Health can be considered a response that pleases God.

Ask your group to identify how focusing on accomplishments and collecting accolades can take away from their efforts to live a balanced life for Christ.

During Day Six, members will begin to work on their First Place 4 Health testimony. Using Ephesians 2:1-10 as your template, talk to your group about the three elements of testimony.

During the Day Seven reflection and application time, your group was asked to write all of the memory verses they have learned during this session. Have different members say each verse, and then talk about how that verse can be applied to First Place 4 Health. Offer a small prize for group members who can say all seven verses from memory!

week nine: our power supply

In the introduction to this week's study, members read an overview about power that comes from God's Spirit as opposed to the feeling of powerlessness that often characterizes our lives. Have someone in your group who has successfully reached his or her goal weight talk about how the Spirit's power allowed him or her to do what he or she could not have done alone.

Zechariah came to minister to God's people as they rebuilt the Temple. In First Place 4 Health, we are rebuilding God's Temple as well. Talk about how this is a spiritual calling, not just a self-improvement project.

Ask members of your group to identify how First Place 4 Health is calling them to a more intimate relationship with God. Also ask the group to talk about how God has been encouraging them during this session. Try to pick different people to talk this time!

Unless we believe in the truth of God's Word, all our Bible study is to no avail. Stress the important concept of all Scripture being "God-breathed."

Three of the present-day ministries of the Holy Spirit are (1) to convict God's people of sin, (2) to convince God's people of the righteousness of Jesus Christ, and (3) to convince people of the certainty of future judgment. Put these three categories on your whiteboard or flip chart, and then talk about how First Place 4 Health is part of the Spirit's work in each of these areas.

Ask your group to share what they have learned about the Spirit this week. If you are not well versed in the ministry of the Holy Spirit, ask your pastor or a Christian educator to come and talk to your group about the Holy Spirit.

On Day Seven, group members were asked to sit in silence and allow the Holy Spirit to hover over them. Have your group talk about that experience.

The Holy Spirit teaches us to pray! End your session with prayer.

week ten: Jesus paid it all

Most of us can identify with the apostle Paul's struggle with sin. Ask your group members to share their struggle with knowing what to do, but not doing it. It is important that you do not allow this to turn into a discussion about condemnation either on the part of the one talking or of the ones listening.

Have someone in your group read Titus 3:3-5. This will be very similar to what the members studied in Ephesians 2 during Week Seven. Point out the "how it was," "what happened" and "how it is now" elements of this passage.

Ask your group if they have begun to assemble their personal faith stories. Answer any questions they might have about the process at this time.

Many people can quote the first half of Romans 6:23, but very few know that there is a second part! Have your group recite Romans 6:23 in unison. Talk about the free gift of God.

Draw the four-sided person chart that appears in the Day Three study on your whiteboard or flip chart. Talk about how the four parts of our being can be at war with one another when we are not leading a balanced life and walking in sync with the Spirit.

Be sensitive to the feelings the two categories of people will bring up for those who have family members who do not appear to be believers. Stress God's grace and how He waits patiently so that none will perish.

During the Day Seven reflection and application time, your group members made "New Beginnings" collages. Have members share their collages with the group and explain why they chose the items that are on their sheet.

week eleven: trust in the Lord

We are nearing the end of this session of First Place 4 Health. Begin this week's group time by having the members read Proverbs 3:5-8 in unison. Then lead a brief discussion about the importance of trusting God in all things and at all times.

Ask your members to explain the importance of understanding the context in which a particular verse was written.

In Day One, members read how David felt compelled to sing God's praise with his whole heart. Have members share their songs of victory from the Day One study and explain how God has subdued their foes and upheld their cause during this session of First Place 4 Health.

Each time we trust God, He proves Himself faithful and worthy of our trust. Have members discuss what they have trusted to God during this session and how He has proven Himself worthy of that trust.

Lead a short discussion on how being wholehearted in our devotion is synonymous with putting Christ first in all things.

Matthew 6:33, the core verse of First Place 4 Health, tells us to seek God's kingdom and righteousness, and "all these things" will be given to us as well. Have members talk about the blessings they have received from God during this session as they have sought to please Him and do His will.

By now, your group should have completed their final assessment with regard to the goals they set at the beginning of the Bible study. Let them know that they will be sharing their progress and their testimonies as part of next week's victory celebration.

week twelve: time to celebrate!

Even though most of your meeting this week will be a victory celebration, take some time at the beginning of the meeting to talk about how much God loves each person in the group and how each person is called to love their brothers and sisters in Christ. (Refer to "Planning a Victory Celebration" in the *First Place 4 Health Leader's Guide* for some ideas about throwing a successful celebration for your group.)

For the rest of the study time, allow each member to tell his or her *Daily Victory, Daily Joy* story. Give members an equal opportunity to share the goals they set for themselves at the beginning of the session and talk about the challenges and good things God has done for them throughout the process. Don't allow the more talkative group members to monopolize all the time. Even the quiet members need an opportunity to share their stories and successes! Even those who have not met their goals have still been part of the journey, so allow them to share and talk about why they did not succeed.

Making a commitment to continue in First Place 4 Health is an important part of victory. Be sure to talk about your group's future plans, and make each person feel welcome to continue to journey with you.

End your victory celebration by reading Aaron's blessing found in Numbers 6:24-26, which is a wonderful way to conclude this session.

First Place 4 Health
menu plans

Each menu plan is based on approximately 1,400 to 1,500 calories per day. All recipe and menu exchanges were determined using the MasterCook software, a program that accesses a database containing more than 6,000 food items prepared using the United States Department of Agriculture (USDA) publications and information from food manufactuzrers. As with any nutritional program, MasterCook calculates the nutritional values of the recipes based on ingredients. Nutrition may vary due to how the food is prepared, where the food comes from, soil content, season, ripeness, processing and method of preparation. For these reasons, please use the recipes and menu plans as approximate guides. As always, consult your physician and/or a registered dietitian before starting a weight-loss program.

For those who need more calories, add the following to the 1,400-calorie plan:

- 1,800 calories: 2 ounce equivalent of meat, 3 ounce equivalent of bread, $1/2$ cup vegetable serving, 1 tsp. fat

- 2,000 calories: 2 ounce equivalent of meat, 4 ounce equivalent of bread, $1/2$ cup vegetable serving, 3 tsp. fat

- 2,200 calories: 2 ounce equivalent of meat, 5 ounce equivalent of bread, $1/2$ cup vegetable serving, $1/2$ cup fruit serving, 5 tsp. fat

- 2,400 calories: 2 ounce equivalent of meat, 6 ounce equivalent of bread, 1 cup vegetable serving, $1/2$ cup fruit serving, 6 tsp. fat

First Week Grocery List

Produce
- ☐ onions
- ☐ (2) green bell peppers
- ☐ garlic
- ☐ (5) tomatoes
- ☐ (1) green chili pepper
- ☐ 3 cups fresh basil leaves
- ☐ (2) peaches
- ☐ (1) grapefruit
- ☐ (1) container strawberries
- ☐ (1) bunch spinach leaves
- ☐ (1) bunch romaine lettuce
- ☐ (1) bunch broccoli
- ☐ (1) bunch green onions
- ☐ fresh parsley
- ☐ (2) oranges
- ☐ bananas
- ☐ apples
- ☐ (1) zucchini
- ☐ baby carrots
- ☐ pears
- ☐ okra
- ☐ asparagus
- ☐ lemon

Baking Products
- ☐ nonstick cooking spray
- ☐ baking powder
- ☐ baking soda
- ☐ (1) jar applesauce
- ☐ olive oil
- ☐ tomato juice
- ☐ orange juice
- ☐ wheat germ
- ☐ pine nuts
- ☐ walnuts
- ☐ raisins
- ☐ whole-wheat flour
- ☐ nonfat Italian salad dressing or light dressing of choice
- ☐ basil
- ☐ oregano
- ☐ garlic powder
- ☐ pepper
- ☐ salt
- ☐ mustard
- ☐ sugar-free maple syrup
- ☐ reduced-fat Ranch dressing
- ☐ apple juice
- ☐ salsa
- ☐ molasses
- ☐ safflower oil
- ☐ sesame seeds
- ☐ cinnamon
- ☐ peanuts, dry-roasted

Breads and Cereals
- ☐ corn muffins
- ☐ Italian bread
- ☐ whole-wheat sliced bread
- ☐ raisin bread
- ☐ English muffins
- ☐ dinner rolls
- ☐ quick-cooking grits
- ☐ Shredded Wheat®
- ☐ oatmeal
- ☐ Ryvita crackers
- ☐ graham crackers
- ☐ saltine crackers
- ☐ whole-wheat pasta

- brown rice
- (1) pkg. small whole-wheat tortillas

Canned Foods

- (1) 1-lb. can kidney beans
- (1) can mandarin oranges in juice
- (1) can corn
- (1) can Campbell's Chunky Minestrone Soup
- (1) can gazpacho soup
- (2) 16-ounce cans tomato sauce

Dairy Products

- 12-oz. reduced-fat cheddar cheese
- light margarine
- eggs

- 8-oz. part-skim milk mozzarella cheese
- skim milk
- 8-oz. fresh Parmesan cheese
- buttermilk
- cream cheese
- 8-oz. nonfat artificially sweetened vanilla yogurt
- low-fat cottage cheese
- string cheese
- nonfat plain yogurt

Frozen Foods

- frozen cod fillets
- mixed fruit
- Lean Cuisine Café Classic
- Michelina's Roasted Sirloin Supreme Dinner
- Healthy Choice Complete Selection Dinner

First Week Meals and Recipes

DAY 1

Breakfast

$1/2$ cup Shredded Wheat® with
  1 cup skim milk
1 sliced peach

1 slice raisin toast with
  1 tbsp. cream cheese

Nutritional Information: 334 calories; 7g fat (18.2% calories from fat); 14g protein; 57g carbohydrate; 6g dietary fiber; 20mg cholesterol; 272mg sodium.

Lunch

Broiled Open-faced Vegetarian Sandwich

2 slices Italian bread (cut 1" thick)
1 tbsp. reduced-calorie margarine
Zucchini slices
Tomato slices
Onion slices
Green bell pepper slices

Garlic powder
Basil
Pepper
2 oz. part-skim milk
  mozzarella cheese
1 small banana

Spread Italian bread with 1 tsp. reduced-calorie margarine on each. Top with tomato, zucchini, onion and green bell pepper slices. Sprinkle with garlic powder, basil and pepper; top with cheese. Broil until browned on edges and cheese is melted. Serve with 1 small banana. Serves 1.

Nutritional Information: 431 calories; 17g fat (35.3% calories from fat); 21g protein; 51g carbohydrate; 4g dietary fiber; 31mg cholesterol; 674mg sodium.

Dinner

3 oz. frozen cod (baked per package
  instructions) with 2 tbsp. nonfat
  plain yogurt and 1 tsp. mustard
  spread on top before baking
$1/2$ cup asparagus with lemon wedge

$2/3$ cup cooked rice
Tossed salad with 2 tbsp.
  reduced-calorie dressing
$3/4$ cup water-packed mandarin
  orange sections, drained

Nutritional Information: 388 calories; 5g fat (13.2% calories from fat); 10g protein; 64g carbohydrate; 7g dietary fiber; 2mg cholesterol; 476mg sodium.

DAY 2

Breakfast

1 English muffin with
  1 tsp. margarine

1 poached egg
$1/_2$ grapefruit

Nutritional Information: 280 calories; 10g fat (31.8% calories from fat); 11g protein; 36g carbohydrate; 3g dietary fiber; 212mg cholesterol; 449mg sodium.

Lunch

$1/_2$ can Campbell's Chunky
  Minestrone Soup, heated
1 cup mixed greens with
  2 tomato slices
8 saltine crackers

$1/_2$ cup baby carrots with 2 tbsp.
  reduced-fat Ranch dressing
$1/_2$ cup apple juice

Nutritional Information: 325 calories; 7g fat (18.0% calories from fat); 9g protein; 60g carbohydrate; 6g dietary fiber; 3mg cholesterol; 1,294mg sodium.

Dinner

Bean Enchilada

2 tsp. olive oil
$1/_3$ cup finely chopped onions
$1/_3$ cup finely chopped green
  bell pepper
5 cloves garlic, minced
16 oz. tomato sauce

$1/_2$ tsp. basil
$1/_2$ tsp. oregano
1 cup steamed broccoli
$2/_3$ cup cooked brown rice

Filling:

2 tsp. olive oil
1 cup chopped onions
4 cloves garlic, minced
1-lb. can kidney beans, about
  3 cups, mashed
1 green bell pepper, chopped

1 cup canned or frozen corn, drained
8 whole-wheat tortillas
3 oz. (about $3/_4$ cup) shredded
  low-fat cheddar cheese

To make sauce, sauté onions, green bell pepper, and garlic in oil. Cook until tender, about 5 minutes. Remove from heat and add remaining sauce ingredients; set aside. For filling, sauté onions, green bell pepper, and garlic for about 5 minutes. Add mashed kidney beans, corn, and $^1/_2$ cup sauce. To assemble enchiladas, spread $^1/_2$ cup sauce on the bottom of a 6 × 10-inch baking pan. Spread $^1/_3$ cup of bean mixture onto each tortilla. Roll up tightly and place tortillas in pan seam side down. Spoon remaining sauce over tortillas. Cover and bake in the oven at 350°F for 30 minutes. Uncover, sprinkle with cheese, and then bake for 5 more minutes. Serve one bean enchilada with 1 cup steamed broccoli and $^2/_3$ cup cooked brown rice. Serves 8.

Nutritional Information: 593 calories; 10g fat (15.3% calories from fat); 24g protein; 105g carbohydrate; 17g dietary fiber; 2mg cholesterol; 804mg sodium.

DAY 3

Breakfast

1 cup oatmeal with dash of cinnamon and brown sugar substitute, if desired
1 tbsp. raisins

$^1/_4$ cup applesauce
1 cup skim milk

Nutritional Information: 299 calories; 3g fat (8.6% calories from fat); 15g protein; 56g carbohydrate; 5g dietary fiber; 4mg cholesterol; 506mg sodium.

Lunch

Taco Bell Light Chicken Burrito
1 cup gazpacho soup

1 small apple

Nutritional Information: 538 calories; 16g fat (26.2% calories from fat); 24g protein; 75g carbohydrate; 8g dietary fiber; 55mg cholesterol; 2,119mg sodium.

Dinner

1 Healthy Choice Complete Selection Dinner
1 small dinner roll with 1 tsp. margarine

Spinach salad with $^1/_2$ hard-boiled egg, chopped, and 2 tbsp. reduced calorie salad dressing

Nutritional Information: 578 calories; 18g fat (28.0% calories from fat); 21g protein; 82g carbohydrate; 8g dietary fiber; 133mg cholesterol; 962mg sodium.

DAY 4

....

Breakfast

French Toast

1 tbsp. reduced-fat or 1 tsp.
  regular margarine and 2 tbsp.
  sugar-free maple syrup, if desired

¹/₂ cup unsweetened applesauce
  with dash of cinnamon
1 cup skim milk

Dip 2 slices of bread in a beaten egg. Brown on both sides in pan sprayed with nonstick cooking spray. Serve with margarine and sugar-free pancake syrup (if desired) and unsweetened applesauce. Serves 1.

Nutritional Information: 395 calories; 13g fat (29.3% calories from fat); 19g protein; 51g carbohydrate; 3g dietary fiber; 217mg cholesterol; 606mg sodium.

....

Lunch

1 oz. package dry-roasted peanuts
2 tubes string cheese
8 Ryvita crackers

4 oz. tomato juice
1 medium apple or pear

Nutritional Information: 469 calories; 20g fat (37.5% calories from fat); 25g protein; 50g carbohydrate; 12g dietary fiber; 20mg cholesterol; 998mg sodium.

....

Dinner

2 slices Pizza Hut Fit-n-Delicious
  Pizza (14″)

Tossed salad with 1 tbsp. salad dressing
¹/₂ cup fresh mixed fruit

Nutritional Information: 573 calories; 14g fat (20.3% calories from fat); 26g protein; 97g carbohydrate; 8g dietary fiber; 41mg cholesterol; 1,790mg sodium.

DAY 5

....

Breakfast

Cheesy Grits

2 cups water
¹/₂ cup quick-cooking grits
³/₄ cup shredded reduced-
  fat cheddar cheese
2 tbsp. chopped green chiles or
  picante sauce

1 egg, separated
¹/₄ cup skim milk
Nonstick cooking spray
¹/₂ grapefruit
1 tbsp. reduced-fat margarine

Preheat oven to 350° F. Bring water to boil in heavy saucepan. Stir in grits. Return to boil, and then reduce heat, partially cover, and cook for 5 minutes. Stir occasionally. Add cheese a little at a time until it melts. Add margarine and chiles or picante sauce. Stir well. Beat egg yolk with milk and stir into grits. Whip egg white until stiff, and then fold into grits. Pour into a 5×5-inch casserole dish sprayed with nonstick cooking spray. Bake 45 minutes until you can insert a knife into the grits and it comes out clean. Remove from oven and let stand 5 minutes before cutting. Serve with ¹/₂ grapefruit. Serves 2.

Nutritional Information: 332 calories; 9g fat (24.2% calories from fat); 19g protein; 34g carbohydrate; 1g dietary fiber; 115mg cholesterol; 387mg sodium.

Lunch
Lean Cuisine Café Classic
1 orange

Nutritional Information: 322 calories; 5g fat (13.8% calories from fat); 18g protein; 54g carbohydrate; 6g dietary fiber; 50mg cholesterol; 690mg sodium.

Dinner

Michelina's Roasted Sirloin
  Supreme Dinner
¹/₂ cup cooked carrots
2 pear halves

1 small corn muffin with
  1 tsp. margarine
¹/₄ cup low-fat cottage cheese

Nutritional Information: 616 calories; 22g fat (31.4% calories from fat); 25g protein; 83g carbohydrate; 8g dietary fiber; 32mg cholesterol; 1,821mg sodium.

DAY 6

Breakfast
McDonald's Egg McMuffin
6 oz. orange juice

Nutritional Information: 377 calories; 12g fat (29.3% calories from fat); 19g protein; 48g carbohydrate; 2g dietary fiber; 260mg cholesterol; 822mg sodium.

Lunch

Pizza Muffins

1 egg	2 tsp. baking powder
$^1/_2$ cup tomato sauce	1 tsp. baking soda
1 cup buttermilk or plain low-fat yogurt	Sliced tomatoes and sesame seeds for garnish
1 tsp. dried oregano	Nonstick vegetable cooking spray
$^1/_4$ tsp. garlic powder	Tossed salad with 2 tbsp. reduced calorie salad dressing
$^1/_4$ tsp. freshly ground pepper	1 apple
4 oz. mozzarella cheese, diced	3 tbsp. wheat germ
$1^1/_2$ cups whole-wheat flour	

Preheat oven to 400° F. Spray muffin tin with nonstick vegetable cooking spray or line with baking cups. Blend the egg, tomato sauce and buttermilk or yogurt with a mixer or food processor. Add the spices. Add the cheese, reserving $^1/_4$ cup for topping. In another bowl, mix the flour, wheat germ, baking powder and baking soda. Combine the two mixtures until flour is no longer visible. Spoon batter into muffin tin, filling each about $^2/_3$ full. Top each muffin with a slice of tomato and some cheese; sprinkle with sesame seeds. Bake 20 to 25 minutes. Serve with tossed salad and 1 apple. Serves 6.

Nutritional Information: 365 calories; 11g fat (24.9% calories from fat); 15g protein; 59g carbohydrate; 11g dietary fiber; 55mg cholesterol; 906mg sodium.

Dinner

1 Taco Bell chicken fajita	1 medium peach or apple
3 tbsp. salsa	

Nutritional Information: 526 calories; 22g fat (37.5% calories from fat); 18g protein; 65g carbohydrate; 7g dietary fiber; 60mg cholesterol; 1,501mg sodium.

DAY 7

Breakfast

Breakfast Delight
Alternate ingredients by layering in parfait dish:

1 graham cracker, $1^1/_2$-inch square, crumbled	8 oz. nonfat artificially sweetened vanilla yogurt

4 walnut halves, chopped
$^1/_2$ cup strawberries, sliced, or
  $^1/_2$ cup blueberries

3 tbsp. wheat germ or
  2 tbsp. bran cereal

Nutritional Information: 345 calories; 11g fat (26.8% calories from fat); 19g protein; 47g carbo-hydrate; 7g dietary fiber; 3mg cholesterol; 219mg sodium.

Lunch

1 Arby's regular roast beef sandwich
1 orange

Tossed salad with 2-3 tbsp. fat-free
  salad dressing

Nutritional Information: 564 calories; 22g fat (33.0% calories from fat); 26g protein; 73g carbo-hydrate; 9g dietary fiber; 39mg cholesterol; 1,596mg sodium.

Dinner

Pasta with Pesto Sauce

2 cloves garlic
1 tsp. salt
3 cups packed basil leaves
2 tbsp. chopped parsley
2 tbsp. pine nuts
$^1/_2$ cup olive oil
$^1/_2$ cup finely grated fresh
  Parmesan cheese
2 tbsp. hot cooking liquid

1 cup whole-wheat pasta
$^1/_2$ cup okra and tomatoes, stewed
1 *Whole Grain Muffin* (see recipe below)
1 cup spinach salad topped with
  1 tbsp. pine nuts and 1 tbsp.
  fat-free dressing

Put the garlic, salt, basil leaves, chopped parsley, olive oil and 2 tbsp. pine nuts in a blender. Blend, pushing down with a rubber spatula until mixture is thoroughly pureed. Beat in the cheese. Add 2 tbsp. of the hot cooking liquid from pasta to the sauce before mixing it with the pasta. Serving size: 2 tbsp. Serve over 1 cup cooked whole-wheat pasta along with $^1/_2$ cup okra and tomatoes, stewed, 1 *Whole-Grain Muffin*, and 1 cup spinach salad topped with 1 tbsp. pine nuts and 1 tbsp. fat-free dressing. Serves 8.

Whole-Grain Muffin

1 cup whole-wheat flour
1 rounded tsp. baking powder
$^1/_2$ tsp. salt
1 tbsp. safflower oil

1 egg, beaten
1 cup buttermilk
1 tbsp. molasses

Preheat oven to 450° F. Mix dry ingredients. Work in oil with pastry blender. Add beaten egg, buttermilk and molasses, and stir well. Fill oiled muffin tins a little more than half full. Bake for 17 minutes. Serves 12.

Nutritional Information: 512 calories; 25g fat (41.7% calories from fat); 18g protein; 61g carbohydrate; 10g dietary fiber; 23mg cholesterol; 677mg sodium.

Second Week Grocery List

Produce
- ❑ onions
- ❑ green bell peppers
- ❑ garlic
- ❑ lemon juice
- ❑ green onions
- ❑ tomatoes
- ❑ broccoli
- ❑ yellow squash
- ❑ red bell peppers
- ❑ fresh ginger
- ❑ kiwi fruits
- ❑ strawberries
- ❑ grapefruits
- ❑ bananas
- ❑ apples
- ❑ cantaloupes
- ❑ fresh parsley
- ❑ spinach leaves
- ❑ peaches
- ❑ corn on the cob
- ❑ asparagus
- ❑ lemon
- ❑ celery
- ❑ grapes
- ❑ oranges
- ❑ baby carrots
- ❑ cilantro
- ❑ lettuce
- ❑ cucumbers
- ❑ green beans
- ❑ raspberries
- ❑ blueberries
- ❑ mushrooms
- ❑ zucchini
- ❑ potatoes
- ❑ plums
- ❑ light firm tofu

Baking Products
- ❑ mustard
- ❑ olive oil
- ❑ Canola oil
- ❑ sugar
- ❑ baking powder
- ❑ $1/2$ lb. dried black beans
- ❑ all-purpose flour
- ❑ cornstarch
- ❑ dill pickle spears
- ❑ spaghetti
- ❑ salsa
- ❑ walnuts
- ❑ almonds
- ❑ wheat germ
- ❑ peanut butter
- ❑ cumin
- ❑ dried oregano
- ❑ dry mustard
- ❑ garlic powder
- ❑ nutmeg
- ❑ salt
- ❑ freshly ground pepper
- ❑ sugar-free fruit spread (strawberry or raspberry)
- ❑ non-stick cooking spray
- ❑ light mayonnaise
- ❑ graham cracker crumb pie crusts
- ❑ orange juice
- ❑ (2) packages artificial sweetener
- ❑ light salad dressing of choice

Breads and Cereals
- ❑ whole-wheat bread
- ❑ whole-wheat English muffins
- ❑ cornbread
- ❑ French bread loaf
- ❑ bread sticks
- ❑ dinner rolls
- ❑ saltine crackers
- ❑ tortillas (small)
- ❑ blueberry bagel
- ❑ instant apple-cinnamon oatmeal
- ❑ Wasa crackers

Canned Foods
- ❑ (1) can peas
- ❑ (1) can mandarin oranges in water
- ❑ (1) can condensed chicken broth
- ❑ (1) can fruit cocktail
- ❑ (1) can vegetable soup
- ❑ (1) can whole tomatoes

Dairy Products
- ❑ eggs
- ❑ skim milk
- ❑ 12-oz. part-skim milk mozzarella cheese
- ❑ American cheese slices
- ❑ 8 oz. Parmesan cheese
- ❑ Monterey jack cheese
- ❑ reduced-fat cheddar cheese
- ❑ 8 oz. nonfat yogurt with fruit, artificial sweetener
- ❑ light margarine
- ❑ egg substitute
- ❑ Cool Whip Lite®

Frozen Foods
- ❑ (1) pkg. frozen chopped spinach
- ❑ cheese tortellini
- ❑ Stouffer's Lean Cuisine Three-Bean Chili Dinner
- ❑ Stouffer's Lean Cuisine Cheese Cannelloni with Tomato Sauce

Seafood and Meat
- ❑ top round steaks
- ❑ chicken breast halves

Second Week Meals and Recipes

DAY 1

Breakfast

Breakfast Tortilla
$1/_2$ cup egg substitute, scrambled with 2 tbsp. chopped onion and
2 tbsp. chopped green bell pepper and 2 tbsp. salsa, wrapped in
(2) 6-inch soft tortillas
1 kiwi fruit

Nutritional Information: 520 calories; 20g fat (55.9% calories from fat); 15g protein; 20g carbohydrate; 4g dietary fiber; 2mg cholesterol; 385mg sodium.

Lunch

Chicken Salad

2 oz. cooked skinless white chicken, chopped	$1/_2$ cup chilled asparagus spears with lemon wedge
2 tbsp. diced celery	1 dill pickle spear
1 tbsp. reduced-fat salad dressing	15 grapes
1 tbsp. toasted, sliced almonds	12 saltine crackers

Combine chopped chicken, diced celery, sliced almonds, asparagus spears, dill pickle spear and grapes in a bowl and mix in reduced-fat salad dressing. Serve with 12 saltine crackers.

Nutritional Information: 399 calories; 14g fat (31.3% calories from fat); 21g protein; 49g carbohydrate; 4g dietary fiber; 39mg cholesterol; 1,021mg sodium.

Dinner

$1/_2$ baked chicken breast (without skin)	Tossed salad with 2 tbsp. reduced-fat salad dressing
1 small baked potato	$3/_4$ cup drained mandarin oranges
$1/_2$ cup peas	Raw vegetable relish tray
1 tsp. margarine	

Nutritional Information: 554 calories; 11g fat (17.1% calories from fat); 38g protein; 79g carbohydrate; 13g dietary fiber; 74mg cholesterol; 393mg sodium.

DAY 2

Breakfast

1 blueberry bagel with 1$^1/_2$ tbsp. reduced-calorie cream cheese

1$^1/_4$ cups fresh strawberries
1 cup skim milk

Nutritional Information: 312 calories; 6g fat (15.7% calories from fat); 16g protein; 50g carbohydrate; 5g dietary fiber; 16mg cholesterol; 485mg sodium.

Lunch

Black Bean Soup

$^1/_2$ lb. dried black beans, rinsed and picked over
1 qt. water
1 tbsp. olive oil
1 cup chopped onions
$^1/_2$ cup chopped green bell pepper
1 tbsp. minced garlic
$^1/_2$ tsp. cumin

$^1/_2$ tsp. dried oregano
$^1/_4$ tsp. dry mustard
1 tbsp. lemon juice
2 tbsp. minced green onion
6 saltine crackers
Tossed salad with 2 tbsp. reduced-fat salad dressing
$^1/_2$ cup unsweetened canned fruit cocktail

Soak beans in water in a large pot for at least 8 hours or overnight (place in refrigerator to soak). After soaking, drain beans and place them in 1 qt. fresh water. Bring to a boil, lower heat, cover, and simmer for 2 hours until beans are tender. Heat oil in saucepan over medium high heat. Add onions and sauté for 5 minutes. Add green bell pepper and sauté for another 3 minutes. Add remaining ingredients. Add about $^3/_4$ cup hot liquid from the simmering beans; cover and simmer onion mixture for 10 minutes. Add onion mixture to beans and continue to cook for 1 hour. To serve, top with minced green onions. Serve with 6 saltine crackers, tossed salad and $^1/_2$ cup unsweetened canned fruit cocktail. Serves 4.

Nutritional Information: 438 calories; 10g fat (19.8% calories from fat); 18g protein; 74g carbohydrate; 15g dietary fiber; 2mg cholesterol; 527mg sodium.

Dinner

Crustless Spinach Quiche

(1) 10-oz. package frozen chopped spinach, thawed and well drained

1 cup shredded part-skim mozzarella cheese

4 eggs, plus 2 egg whites, lightly beaten (or 1¹/₂ cups egg substitute)
1 tbsp. minced onion
¹/₄ tsp. nutmeg
Fresh ground pepper and salt to taste
Nonstick cooking spray

(2) 3-inch slices French bread
1 cup cooked carrots
2 tsp. margarine
Tossed salad with 2 tbsp. reduced-fat salad dressing
1 cup cantaloupe cubes

Preheat oven to 350° F. Combine spinach, eggs, onion, nutmeg, mozzarella cheese and salt and pepper in a medium bowl. Mix well. Transfer mixture to 8-inch pie plate sprayed with nonstick cooking spray. Bake 30 minutes or until you can insert a knife into the quiche and it comes out clean. Remove from oven and let stand 5 minutes; then slice into wedges. Serve with 2 slices French bread, 1 cup cooked carrots, tossed salad and 1 cup cantaloupe cubes. Serves 6.

Nutritional Information: 522 calories; 20g fat (33.2% calories from fat); 22g protein; 69g carbohydrate; 13g dietary fiber; 153mg cholesterol; 986mg sodium.

DAY 3

Breakfast

Peanut Butter and Jelly Muffin
2 cups flour
3 tbsp. sugar
1 tbsp. baking powder
³/₄ cup creamy peanut butter
1 large egg
1 cup low-fat milk

¹/₃ cup sugar-free fruit spread (strawberry or raspberry)
Nonstick vegetable cooking spray
1 cup nonfat fruit-flavored yogurt
¹/₂ grapefruit

Preheat oven to 350° F. Spray muffin tin with nonstick vegetable cooking spray or line with baking cups. In a large bowl, mix flour, sugar and baking powder. In another bowl, beat peanut butter and egg until smooth. Add milk a little at a time, stirring after each addition. Pour peanut butter mixture over dry ingredients; fold in just until dry ingredients are moistened. Batter will be stiff. Spoon 2 scant tbsp. batter into each muffin cup and smooth the surface out to the top edge of the cup. Top each muffin with a heaping tsp. of fruit spread; cover with 2 more tbsp. of batter. Bake 20 to 25 minutes or until lightly browned. Serve with 1 cup nonfat fruit-flavored yogurt and ¹/₂ grapefruit. Serves 12.

Nutritional Information: 353 calories; 10g fat (23.5% calories from fat); 18g protein; 52g carbohydrate; 4g dietary fiber; 22mg cholesterol; 345mg sodium.

Lunch

$1/_2$ Chicken Sandwich

1 slice whole-wheat bread with
  2 oz. chicken breast and
  1 tsp. mayonnaise and lettuce,
  tomato and mustard, as desired

1 orange
1 cup vegetable soup

Nutritional Information: 303 calories; 9g fat (24.7% calories from fat); 19g protein; 40g carbohydrate; 6g dietary fiber; 36mg cholesterol; 1,025mg sodium.

Dinner

(1) 9-oz. Wendy's chili
Tossed salad with 2 tbsp. reduced-
  calorie Italian dressing

6 saltine crackers
1 peach

Nutritional Information: 362 calories; 12g fat (30.0% calories from fat); 17g protein; 46g carbohydrate; 8g dietary fiber; 32mg cholesterol; 1,270mg sodium.

DAY 4

Breakfast

1 package instant apple-cinnamon oatmeal with 4 walnut halves,
  chopped, and $1/_2$ banana
1 cup skim milk

Nutritional Information: 352 calories; 9g fat (22.4% calories from fat); 18g protein; 53g carbohydrate; 6g dietary fiber; 4mg cholesterol; 536mg sodium.

Lunch

Tomato-cheese Bake Sandwich

2 slices whole-wheat bread
2 slices American cheese
4 slices tomato
6 green bell pepper strips

1 tbsp. reduced-calorie salad dressing
15 grapes

Top each slice of bread with 2 slices of tomato, 3 strips of green bell pepper and half of the salad dressing. Place 1 slice of cheese over the dressing and sprinkle with oregano. Broil until cheese is melted. Serve with 15 grapes. Serves 2.

Nutritional Information: 492 calories; 23g fat (39.8% calories from fat); 22g protein; 56g carbohydrate; 10g dietary fiber; 54mg cholesterol, 1,269mg sodium.

Dinner

Stouffer's Lean Cuisine
  Three-Bean Chili Dinner
2-inch square corn bread

1 large tomato
$^1/_2$ cucumber, sliced
1 cup skim milk

Nutritional Information: 526 calories; 13g fat (19.7% calories from fat); 24g protein; 92g carbohydrate; 11g dietary fiber; 40mg cholesterol; 1,188mg sodium.

DAY 5

Breakfast

6 Wasa crackers with
  1 oz. cheddar cheese
1 medium apple

Nutritional Information: 331 calories; 10g fat (25.6% calories from fat); 13g protein; 51g carbohydrate; 10g dietary fiber; 30mg cholesterol; 416mg sodium.

Lunch

1 piece Kentucky Fried Chicken
  skinless center breast
1 ear corn-on-the-cob

1 medium apple
1 serving coleslaw

Nutritional Information: 382 calories; 7g fat (14.6% calories from fat); 34g protein; 54g carbohydrate; 8g dietary fiber; 75mg cholesterol; 561mg sodium.

Dinner

Chicken Fried Steak with Pan Gravy

1 lb. boneless top round steak
  pounded to $^1/_3$-inch thickness
1 egg
1 tbsp. water
$^1/_2$ tsp. garlic powder
Fresh ground pepper and salt to taste
$^1/_4$ cup all-purpose flour

Nonstick cooking spray
$1^1/_2$ tbsp. canola oil
$^3/_4$ cup mashed potatoes
1 cup green beans
2 tsp. margarine
1 orange

Gravy
2 tbsp. all-purpose flour
$1/_2$ cup water
$1/_2$ cup skim milk

Cut fat from steak and cut into four pieces. Beat egg with water for about 2 minutes until lemon-colored. Combine seasonings and sprinkle on both sides of steak. Dredge each piece of steak in flour and shake off excess, then dip in egg and again in flour. Spray a large skillet with nonstick cooking spray. Add oil and heat on medium high. Add steak pieces and brown both sides of meat, turning once, for a total of 8 minutes. Reduce heat to low. Cook for 10 to 15 minutes until juices run clear. Remove steak and put on a heated plate. Add 2 tbsp. flour to pan drippings; when light brown, stir in water and milk, whisking until it thickens into a gravy. Add more water if gravy is too thick. Return steaks to skillet; simmer gently until ready to serve. Serve with $3/_4$ cup mashed potatoes, 1 cup green beans, dinner roll and 1 orange. Serves 4.

Nutritional Information: 687 calories; 30g fat (39.2% calories from fat); 37g protein; 69g carbohydrate; 11g dietary fiber; 110mg cholesterol; 702mg sodium.

DAY 6

Breakfast

$1/_2$ English muffin, toasted, with
   1 tbsp. peanut butter and
   $1/_2$ banana
1 cup skim milk

Nutritional Information: 302 calories; 9g fat (27.1% calories from fat); 15g protein; 42g carbohydrate; 3g dietary fiber; 4mg cholesterol; 334mg sodium.

Lunch

Tortilla Soup
(3) 6-inch flour tortillas,
   cut in $1/_2$-inch strips
(1) 4 oz. can whole tomatoes
$1/_2$ small onion, chopped
$1/_2$ clove garlic, chopped
2 cups chicken broth
$1/_4$ tsp. salt

1 tbsp. cilantro
2 tbsp. Monterey Jack cheese, shredded
Nonstick vegetable cooking spray
Tossed salad with 2 tbsp. reduced-
   calorie salad dressing
2 small plums

Fry tortilla strips in heated skillet that has been well coated with nonstick vegetable cooking spray. Puree tomatoes, onions and garlic. Bring chicken broth to a boil in a 2-quart saucepan. Stir in tomato puree, salt and cilantro. Reduce heat and simmer for 10 minutes. Add half of the tortilla strips to soup. Garnish with cheese and remaining tortilla strips to serve. Serve with tossed salad and 2 small plums. Serves 2.

Nutritional Information: 433 calories; 13g fat (38.5% calories from fat); 11g protein; 34g carbohydrate; 7g dietary fiber; 8mg cholesterol; 1,352mg sodium.

Dinner

Vegetable Stir Fry

1 red bell pepper, thinly sliced
1 cup broccoli florets
1 small onion, quartered
1 cup cooked cold spaghetti
1 lb. tofu, cubed
2 tbsp. olive oil

$^{1}/_{2}$ tbsp. fresh ginger, grated
8 oz. Parmesan cheese
1 serving *Light and Creamy Yogurt Pie*
 (see Dessert Recipes) with 2 tbsp.
 raspberry sauce

Heat nonstick skillet or wok to medium high. Add oil and onion and stir 2 minutes. Add pepper and stir 1 minute more. Add ginger, broccoli and tofu and stir 2 minutes more. Add spaghetti and stir until mixture is thoroughly heated. Top each serving with 2 oz. Parmesan cheese. Serve each with one serving *Light and Creamy Yogurt Pie* with 2 tbsp. raspberry sauce (blend 1 cup raspberries with 2 tbsp. orange juice and 2 packets artificial sweetener). Serves 4.

Nutritional Information: 631 calories; 34g fat (47.2% calories from fat); 39g protein; 46g carbohydrate; 6g dietary fiber; 45mg cholesterol; 1,286mg sodium.

DAY 7

Breakfast

Vegetable Frittata

2 whole eggs
4 egg whites
2 oz. low-fat cheese, shredded
1 medium green bell pepper,
 cut in strips
1 medium yellow squash, thinly sliced

1 small onion, thinly sliced
2 tsp. olive oil
Nonstick vegetable cooking spray
1 whole-wheat English muffin with
 2 tsp. light margarine
$^{1}/_{4}$ medium cantaloupe

Preheat oven to 350° F. Whisk eggs with egg whites and set aside. Spray medium saucepan with nonstick vegetable cooking spray. Add oil. Sauté vegetables for 5-7 minutes over medium-high heat. Place sautéed vegetables into a baking dish sprayed with nonstick vegetable cooking spray. Pour blended eggs onto sautéed vegetables and sprinkle cheese on top. Bake frittata for 12-15 minutes (or keep in sauté pan and cook on stovetop over low heat for 10-12 minutes). Serve with 1 whole-wheat English muffin and $1/4$ medium cantaloupe. Serves 4.

Nutritional Information: 338 calories; 11g fat (29.0% calories from fat); 18g protein; 45g carbohydrate; 7g dietary fiber; 109mg cholesterol; 703mg sodium.

Lunch

Stouffer's Lean Cuisine Cheese Cannelloni with Tomato Sauce
$1/2$ cup steamed broccoli with 1 tsp. regular margarine

2 bread sticks
1 cup mixed berries (strawberries, raspberries, blueberries)

Nutritional Information: 350 calories; 11g fat (29.2% calories from fat); 12g protein; 45g carbohydrate; 7g dietary fiber; 20mg cholesterol; 826mg sodium.

Dinner

Tortellini Primavera
$1/2$ cup frozen cheese tortellini
$1/3$ cup each broccoli, mushrooms, zucchini and asparagus, chunked or sliced
$1/2$ small clove garlic, minced
$1/2$ tsp. olive oil
$1/2$ cup skim milk
1 tsp. cornstarch

Pinch nutmeg
Freshly ground pepper
2 tbsp. sliced green onion
1 tbsp. parsley
2 tbsp. Parmesan cheese
Tossed green salad with 1 tbsp. fat-free dressing
$1/2$ cup skim or 1% milk

Boil water and cook tortellini according to package directions while proceeding with the vegetables. Sauté vegetables and garlic in nonstick skillet with oil on medium-high heat for about 1 minute. Reduce heat and cover for 1 to 2 more minutes until tender crisp. Remove cover and add the combination of milk and cornstarch. Stir constantly until thickened. Add nutmeg and pepper to taste. Toss together with tortellini, parsley and green onion. Sprinkle with Parmesan cheese. Serve with tossed green salad with 1 tbsp. fat-free dressing and $1/2$ cup skim or 1% milk. Serves 1.

Nutritional Information: 316 calories; 9g fat (24.1% calories from fat); 22g protein; 39g carbohydrate; 4g dietary fiber; 42mg cholesterol; 731mg sodium.

HEALTHY SNACK OPTIONS

(**Note**: You will need to add the ingredients for these items to the grocery lists.)

Frosty Grapes
1 lb. seedless grapes
(1) 3-oz. package of lime sugar-free gelatin powder

Divide grapes into small bunches. Rinse and drain. Put gelatin powder in a container with a lid that can be frozen. Add grapes and shake to coat. Shake off excess powder from grape bunches. Put lid on container and freeze. Serve frozen. Serves 4.

Nutritional Information: 130 calories; trace fat (1.3% calories from fat); 9g protein; 12g carbohydrate; 1g dietary fiber; 0mg cholesterol; 560mg sodium.

Spicy Strawberries with Balsamic Vinegar
1 1/2 cups strawberries, hulled
    and sliced
1 tbsp. balsamic vinegar
1 tsp. Splenda
1/2 tsp. freshly ground black pepper

Combine all ingredients. Cover and refrigerate until ready to serve.

Nutritional Information: 72 calories; 1g fat (8.5% calories from fat); 1g protein; 17g carbohydrate; 5g dietary fiber; 0mg cholesterol; 3mg sodium.

Vegetable Salsa
1 cup diced zucchini
1 cup chopped red onion
2 red bell peppers, seeded
    and diced
2 green bell peppers, seeded
    and diced
4 tomatoes, diced
2 garlic cloves, minced
1/2 cup chopped fresh cilantro
1 tsp. ground black pepper
2 tsp. sugar
1/4 cup lime juice
1 tsp. salt
Baked pita chips or baked
    corn chips

Wash vegetables and prepare as directed. In a large bowl, combine all the ingredients. Toss gently to mix. Cover and refrigerate for at least 30 minutes to allow the flavors to blend. Great with baked pita chips or baked corn chips.

Nutritional Information per 1/2 cup serving: 20 calories; no fat; 1g protein; 5g carbohydrate; 1g dietary fiber; 0mg cholesterol; 150mg sodium.

Sweet & Spicy Snack Mix

2 cans (15 oz. each) garbanzos, rinsed, drained and patted dry
2 cups Wheat Chex cereal
1 cup dried pineapple chunks
1 cup raisins
2 tbsp. honey
Butter-flavored cooking spray

2 tbsp. reduced-sodium Worcestershire sauce
1 tsp. garlic powder
1/2 tsp. chili powder

Preheat the oven to 350° F. Lightly coat a 15 1/2 × 10 1/2-inch baking sheet with butter-flavored cooking spray. Generously spray a heavy skillet with butter-flavored cooking spray. Add garbanzos to the skillet and cook over medium heat, stirring frequently until the beans begin to brown, about 10 minutes. Transfer garbanzos to the prepared baking sheet. Spray the beans lightly with cooking spray. Bake, stirring frequently, until the beans are crisp, about 20 minutes. Lightly coat a roasting pan with butter-flavored cooking spray. Measure the cereal, pineapple and raisins into the pan. Add roasted garbanzos. Stir to mix evenly. Combine honey, Worcestershire sauce and spices in a large glass measuring cup. Stir to mix evenly. Pour the mixture over the snack mix and toss gently. Spray mixture again with cooking spray. Bake for about 10 to 15 minutes, stirring occasionally to keep the mixture from burning. Remove from oven and let cool. Store in an airtight container.

Nutritional Information per 1/2 cup serving: 154 calories; trace fat; 3g protein; 36g carbohydrate; 3g dietary fiber; 0mg cholesterol; 192mg sodium.

Apples with Sweet & Creamy Dip

8 oz. fat-free cream cheese
2 tbsp. brown sugar
1 1/2 tsp. vanilla
2 tbsp. chopped peanuts

1/2 cup orange juice
4 apples, cored and sliced

Place the cream cheese on the counter for about 5 minutes to allow it to soften. To make the dip, combine the brown sugar, vanilla and cream cheese in a small bowl. Mix until smooth. Stir in the chopped peanuts. Place the apples in another bowl. Drizzle orange juice over the apples to prevent browning. Serve the sliced apples with the dip. Serves 4.

Nutritional Information: 177 calories; 3g fat; 1g saturated sat; 10g protein; 28g carbohydrate; 4g dietary fiber; 4mg cholesterol; 326mg sodium.

DESSERT RECIPES

(**Note**: You will need to add the ingredients for these items to the grocery lists.)

Raspberry Fudge Brownie

(1) 10-oz. package of frozen raspberries in light syrup, thawed but not drained
1/4 cup plus 2 tbsp. margarine
1/4 cup plus 2 tbsp. unsweetened cocoa
1/2 cup sugar
2 eggs, beaten
1/2 tsp. vanilla
1 1/2 cups flour
1/8 tsp. salt

Drain raspberries, reserving 3 tbsp. juice. Set raspberries and juice aside. Combine margarine and cocoa in a large saucepan. Cook over low heat, stirring constantly, until margarine melts and mixture becomes smooth. Remove from heat and let cool slightly. Add sugar, eggs and vanilla to cocoa mixture, stirring well. Combine flour and salt and add to cocoa mixture, folding in gently. Gently fold raspberries into cocoa mixture. Spoon batter into an 8-inch square baking dish that has been coated with nonstick vegetable cooking spray. Bake at 350° F for 20 minutes or until toothpick comes out clean. Cut into 20 squares. Serves 20.

Nutritional Information: 112 calories; 4g fat (33.2% calories from fat); 2g protein; 17g carbohydrate; 1g dietary fiber; 21mg cholesterol; 61mg sodium.

Light and Creamy Yogurt Pie

1 package low-fat whipped topping (equal to 8 oz. or 1 cup)
1 cup nonfat yogurt with artificial sweetener
2 cups sliced strawberries or 1 1/2 cups other fruit
1 store-bought graham cracker crust

Make whipped topping according to package directions. Fold in yogurt and most of the fruit. Fill crust. Garnish with remaining fruit. Chill or freeze. May be served frozen. Serves 8.

Nutritional Information: 173 calories; 8g fat (38.3% calories from fat); 3g protein; 25g carbohydrate; 2g dietary fiber; trace cholesterol; 188mg sodium.

Baked Apple

1 baking apple (Rome, Jonathan, or Granny Smith)
1/2 can diet lemon-lime soda
1/4 tsp. cinnamon
1/2 tbsp. raisins

Preheat oven to 350° F. Core apple without cutting all the way through to the bottom. Peel one strip of skin around the top of the apple. Place apple in a small casserole dish sprayed with nonstick cooking spray. Sprinkle the cavity with cinnamon and stuff with raisins. Pour soda over apple. Bake uncovered for 20 to 30 minutes until apple is soft. Serves 1.

Nutritional Information: 96 calories; 1g fat (4.5% calories from fat); trace protein; 25g carbohydrate; 4g dietary fiber; 0mg cholesterol; 3mg sodium.

Member Survey

Please answer the following questions to help your leader plan your First Place 4 Health meetings so that your needs might be met in this session. Give this form to your leader at the first group meeting.

Name _____   Birth date _____

Please list those who live in your household.

Name   Relationship   Age
_____   _____   _____
_____   _____   _____
_____   _____   _____
_____   _____   _____
_____   _____   _____

What church do you attend? _____

Are you interested in receiving more information about our church?   ❐ Yes   ❐ No

Occupation: _____

What talent or area of expertise would you be willing to share with our class?

_____

_____

Why did you join First Place 4 Health?

_____

_____

With notice, would you be willing to lead a Bible study discussion one week?   ❐ Yes   ❐ No

Are you comfortable praying out loud?   ❐ Yes   ❐ No

If the assistant leader were absent, would you be willing to assist in weighing in members and possibly evaluating the Live It Trackers?   ❐ Yes   ❐ No

Any other comments:

_____

_____

_____

_____

Personal Weight and Measurement Record

Week	Weight	+ or -	Goal this Session	Pounds to goal
1				
2				
3				
4				
5				
6				
7				
8				
9				
10				
11				
12				

Beginning Measurements

Waist _____ Hips _____ Thighs _____ Chest _____

Ending Measurements

Waist _____ Hips _____ Thighs _____ Chest _____

First Place 4 Health
Prayer Partner Form

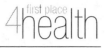

SCRIPTURE VERSE TO MEMORIZE FOR WEEK TWO:
*Now what I am commanding you today is not
too difficult for you or beyond your reach.*
DEUTERONOMY 30:11

Date: _____

Name: _____

Home Phone: (_____) _____

Work Phone: (_____) _____

Email: _____

Personal Prayer Concerns:

_____

_____

_____

_____

_____

_____

_____

This form is for prayer requests that are personal to you and your journey in First Place 4 Health. Please complete this form and have it ready to turn in when you arrive at your group meeting.

First Place 4 Health
Prayer Partner Form

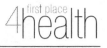

DAILY VICTORY
DAILY JOY
Week
2

Date: _____

Name: _____

Home Phone: (_____) _____

Work Phone: (_____) _____

Email: _____

Personal Prayer Concerns:

_____

_____

_____

_____

_____

_____

_____

This form is for prayer requests that are personal to you and your journey in First Place 4 Health. Please complete this form and have it ready to turn in when you arrive at your group meeting.

First Place 4 Health
Prayer Partner Form

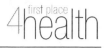

DAILY VICTORY
DAILY JOY
Week
3

SCRIPTURE VERSE TO MEMORIZE FOR WEEK FOUR:
Be self-controlled and alert. Your enemy the devil prowls around like a roaring lion looking for someone to devour.
1 PETER 5:8

Date: _____

Name: _____

Home Phone: (_____) _____

Work Phone: (_____) _____

Email: _____

Personal Prayer Concerns:

_____

_____

_____

_____

_____

_____

_____

This form is for prayer requests that are personal to you and your journey in First Place 4 Health. Please complete this form and have it ready to turn in when you arrive at your group meeting.

First Place 4 Health
Prayer Partner Form

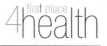

DAILY VICTORY
DAILY JOY
Week
4

Date: _____

Name: _____

Home Phone: (_____) _____

Work Phone: (_____) _____

Email: _____

Personal Prayer Concerns:

_____

_____

_____

_____

_____

_____

_____

This form is for prayer requests that are personal to you and your journey in First Place 4 Health. Please complete this form and have it ready to turn in when you arrive at your group meeting.

First Place 4 Health
Prayer Partner Form

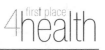

DAILY VICTORY
DAILY JOY
Week
5

SCRIPTURE VERSE TO MEMORIZE FOR WEEK SIX:
*Call to me and I will answer you and tell you great
and unsearchable things you do not know.*
JEREMIAH 33:3

Date: _____

Name: _____

Home Phone: (_____) _____

Work Phone: (_____) _____

Email: _____

Personal Prayer Concerns:

_____

_____

_____

_____

_____

_____

_____

_____

This form is for prayer requests that are personal to you and your journey in First Place 4 Health. Please complete this form and have it ready to turn in when you arrive at your group meeting.

First Place 4 Health
Prayer Partner Form

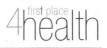

DAILY VICTORY
DAILY JOY
Week
6

SCRIPTURE VERSE TO MEMORIZE FOR WEEK SEVEN:
*We make it our goal to please him, whether we
are at home in the body or away from it.*

2 CORINTHIANS 5:9

Date: _____

Name: _____

Home Phone: (_____)_____

Work Phone: (_____)_____

Email: _____

Personal Prayer Concerns:

_____

_____

_____

_____

_____

_____

_____

This form is for prayer requests that are personal to you and your journey in First Place 4 Health. Please complete this form and have it ready to turn in when you arrive at your group meeting.

First Place 4 Health
Prayer Partner Form

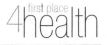

DAILY VICTORY
DAILY JOY
Week
7

Date: _____

Name: _____

Home Phone: (_____) _____

Work Phone: (_____) _____

Email: _____

Personal Prayer Concerns:

_____

_____

_____

_____

_____

_____

_____

This form is for prayer requests that are personal to you and your journey in First Place 4 Health. Please complete this form and have it ready to turn in when you arrive at your group meeting.

First Place 4 Health
Prayer Partner Form

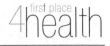

DAILY VICTORY
DAILY JOY
Week
8

"Not by might nor by power, but by my Spirit,"
says the Lord Almighty.
ZECHARIAH 4:6

Date: _____

Name: _____

Home Phone: (_____)_____

Work Phone: (_____)_____

Email: _____

Personal Prayer Concerns:

_____

_____

_____

_____

_____

_____

_____

This form is for prayer requests that are personal to you and your journey in First Place 4 Health. Please complete this form and have it ready to turn in when you arrive at your group meeting.

First Place 4 Health
Prayer Partner Form

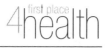

SCRIPTURE VERSE TO MEMORIZE FOR WEEK TEN:
*' Therefore, there is now no condemnation
for those who are in Christ Jesus.*
ROMANS 8:1

Date: _____

Name: _____

Home Phone: (_____)_____

Work Phone: (_____)_____

Email: _____

Personal Prayer Concerns:

_____

_____

_____

_____

_____

_____

_____

This form is for prayer requests that are personal to you and your journey in First Place 4 Health. Please complete this form and have it ready to turn in when you arrive at your group meeting.

First Place 4 Health
Prayer Partner Form

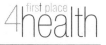

DAILY VICTORY
DAILY JOY
Week
10

SCRIPTURE VERSE TO MEMORIZE FOR WEEK ELEVEN:

*Those who know your name will trust in you, for you,
Lord, have never forsaken those who seek you.*

PSALM 9:10

Date: _____

Name: _____

Home Phone: (_____) _____

Work Phone: (_____) _____

Email: _____

Personal Prayer Concerns:

_____

_____

_____

_____

_____

_____

_____

This form is for prayer requests that are personal to you and your journey in First Place 4 Health. Please complete this form and have it ready to turn in when you arrive at your group meeting.

First Place 4 Health
Prayer Partner Form

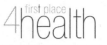

DAILY VICTORY
DAILY JOY
Week
11

Date: _____

Name: _____

Home Phone: (_____) _____

Work Phone: (_____) _____

Email: _____

Personal Prayer Concerns:

_____

_____

_____

_____

_____

_____

_____

This form is for prayer requests that are personal to you and your journey in First Place 4 Health. Please complete this form and have it ready to turn in when you arrive at your group meeting.

Live It Tracker

RECOMMENDED DAILY AMOUNT OF FOOD FROM EACH GROUP

Group	Daily Calories							
	1300-1400	1500-1600	1700-1800	1900 2000	2100-2200	2300-2400	2500-2600	2700-2800
Fruits	1.5-2 c.	1.5-2 c.	1.5-2 c.	2-2.5 c.	2-2.5 c.	2.5-3.5 c.	3.5-4.5 c.	3.5-4.5 c.
Vegetables	1.5-2 c.	2-2.5 c.	2.5-3 c.	2.5-3 c.	3-3.5 c.	3.5-4.5 c.	4.5-5 c.	4.5-5 c.
Grains	5 oz-eq.	5-6 oz-eq.	6-7 oz-eq.	6-7 oz-eq.	7-8 oz-eq.	8-9 oz-eq.	9-10 oz-eq.	10-11 oz-eq.
Meat & Beans	4 oz-eq.	5 oz-eq.	5-5.5 oz-eq.	5.5-6.5 oz-eq.	6.5-7 oz-eq.	7 7.5 oz-eq.	7-7.5 oz-eq.	7.5-8 oz-eq.
Milk	2-3 c.	3 c.	3 c.	3 c.	3 c.	3 c.	3 c.	3 c.
Healthy Oils	4 tsp.	5 tsp.	5 tsp.	6 tsp.	6 tsp.	7 tsp.	8 tsp.	8 tsp.

Day One

FOOD CHOICES

Breakfast: _____ Lunch: _____

Dinner: _____ Snacks: _____

Group	Fruits	Vegetables	Grains	Meat & Beans	Milk	Oils
Goal Amount						
Estimate Your Total						
Increase ⇧ or Decrease ⇩ ?						

PHYSICAL ACTIVITY

Description: _____

Steps/Miles/Minutes: _____

SPIRITUAL ACTIVITY

Description: _____

_____

Day Two

FOOD CHOICES

Breakfast: _____ Lunch: _____

Dinner: _____ Snacks: _____

Group	Fruits	Vegetables	Grains	Meat & Beans	Milk	Oils
Goal Amount						
Estimate Your Total						
Increase ⇧ or Decrease ⇩ ?						

PHYSICAL ACTIVITY

Description: _____

Steps/Miles/Minutes: _____

SPIRITUAL ACTIVITY

Description: _____

_____

Day Three

FOOD CHOICES

Breakfast: _____ Lunch: _____

Dinner: _____ Snacks: _____

Group	Fruits	Vegetables	Grains	Meat & Beans	Milk	Oils
Goal Amount						
Estimate Your Total						
Increase ⇧ or Decrease ⇩ ?						

PHYSICAL ACTIVITY

Description: _____

Steps/Miles/Minutes: _____

SPIRITUAL ACTIVITY

Description: _____

_____

Day Four

FOOD CHOICES

Breakfast: _____ Lunch: _____

Dinner: _____ Snacks: _____

Group	Fruits	Vegetables	Grains	Meat & Beans	Milk	Oils
Goal Amount						
Estimate Your Total						
Increase ⬆ or Decrease ⬇ ?						

PHYSICAL ACTIVITY

Description: _____

Steps/Miles/Minutes: _____

SPIRITUAL ACTIVITY

Description: _____

_____

Day Five

FOOD CHOICES

Breakfast: _____ Lunch: _____

Dinner: _____ Snacks: _____

Group	Fruits	Vegetables	Grains	Meat & Beans	Milk	Oils
Goal Amount						
Estimate Your Total						
Increase ⬆ or Decrease ⬇ ?						

PHYSICAL ACTIVITY

Description: _____

Steps/Miles/Minutes: _____

SPIRITUAL ACTIVITY

Description: _____

_____

Day Six

FOOD CHOICES

Breakfast: _____ Lunch: _____

Dinner: _____ Snacks: _____

Group	Fruits	Vegetables	Grains	Meat & Beans	Milk	Oils
Goal Amount						
Estimate Your Total						
Increase ⬆ or Decrease ⬇ ?						

PHYSICAL ACTIVITY

Description: _____

Steps/Miles/Minutes: _____

SPIRITUAL ACTIVITY

Description: _____

_____

Day Seven

FOOD CHOICES

Breakfast: _____ Lunch: _____

Dinner: _____ Snacks: _____

Group	Fruits	Vegetables	Grains	Meat & Beans	Milk	Oils
Goal Amount						
Estimate Your Total						
Increase ⬆ or Decrease ⬇ ?						

PHYSICAL ACTIVITY

Description: _____

Steps/Miles/Minutes: _____

SPIRITUAL ACTIVITY

Description: _____

_____

Live It Tracker

RECOMMENDED DAILY AMOUNT OF FOOD FROM EACH GROUP

Group	Daily Calories							
	1300-1400	1500-1600	1700-1800	1900-2000	2100-2200	2300-2400	2500-2600	2700-2800
Fruits	1.5-2 c.	1.5-2 c.	1.5-2 c.	2-2.5 c.	2-2.5 c.	2.5-3.5 c.	3.5-4.5 c.	3.5-4.5 c.
Vegetables	1.5-2 c.	2-2.5 c.	2.5-3 c.	2.5-3 c.	3-3.5 c.	3.5-4.5 c.	4.5-5 c.	4.5-5 c.
Grains	5 oz-eq.	5-6 oz-eq.	6-7 oz-eq.	6-7 oz-eq.	7-8 oz-eq.	8-9 oz-eq.	9-10 oz-eq.	10-11 oz-eq.
Meat & Beans	4 oz-eq.	5 oz-eq.	5-5.5 oz-eq.	5.5-6.5 oz-eq.	6.5-7 oz-eq.	7-7.5 oz-eq.	7-7.5 oz-eq.	7.5-8 oz-eq.
Milk	2-3 c.	3 c.	3 c.	3 c.	3 c.	3 c.	3 c.	3 c.
Healthy Oils	4 tsp.	5 tsp.	5 tsp.	6 tsp.	6 tsp.	7 tsp.	8 tsp.	8 tsp.

Day One

FOOD CHOICES

Breakfast: _____   Lunch: _____

Dinner: _____   Snacks: _____

Group	Fruits	Vegetables	Grains	Meat & Beans	Milk	Oils
Goal Amount						
Estimate Your Total						
Increase ⇧ or Decrease ⇩ ?						

PHYSICAL ACTIVITY   **SPIRITUAL ACTIVITY**

Description: _____   Description: _____

Steps/Miles/Minutes: _____

Day Two

FOOD CHOICES

Breakfast: _____   Lunch: _____

Dinner: _____   Snacks: _____

Group	Fruits	Vegetables	Grains	Meat & Beans	Milk	Oils
Goal Amount						
Estimate Your Total						
Increase ⇧ or Decrease ⇩ ?						

PHYSICAL ACTIVITY   **SPIRITUAL ACTIVITY**

Description: _____   Description: _____

Steps/Miles/Minutes: _____

Day Three

FOOD CHOICES

Breakfast: _____   Lunch: _____

Dinner: _____   Snacks: _____

Group	Fruits	Vegetables	Grains	Meat & Beans	Milk	Oils
Goal Amount						
Estimate Your Total						
Increase ⇧ or Decrease ⇩ ?						

PHYSICAL ACTIVITY   **SPIRITUAL ACTIVITY**

Description: _____   Description: _____

Steps/Miles/Minutes: _____

Day Four

FOOD CHOICES

Breakfast: _____ Lunch: _____

Dinner: _____ Snacks: _____

Group	Fruits	Vegetables	Grains	Meat & Beans	Milk	Oils
Goal Amount						
Estimate Your Total						
Increase ⬆ or Decrease ⬇ ?						

PHYSICAL ACTIVITY

Description: _____

Steps/Miles/Minutes: _____

SPIRITUAL ACTIVITY

Description: _____

_____

Day Five

FOOD CHOICES

Breakfast: _____ Lunch: _____

Dinner: _____ Snacks: _____

Group	Fruits	Vegetables	Grains	Meat & Beans	Milk	Oils
Goal Amount						
Estimate Your Total						
Increase ⬆ or Decrease ⬇ ?						

PHYSICAL ACTIVITY

Description: _____

Steps/Miles/Minutes: _____

SPIRITUAL ACTIVITY

Description: _____

_____

Day Six

FOOD CHOICES

Breakfast: _____ Lunch: _____

Dinner: _____ Snacks: _____

Group	Fruits	Vegetables	Grains	Meat & Beans	Milk	Oils
Goal Amount						
Estimate Your Total						
Increase ⬆ or Decrease ⬇ ?						

PHYSICAL ACTIVITY

Description: _____

Steps/Miles/Minutes: _____

SPIRITUAL ACTIVITY

Description: _____

_____

Day Seven

FOOD CHOICES

Breakfast: _____ Lunch: _____

Dinner: _____ Snacks: _____

Group	Fruits	Vegetables	Grains	Meat & Beans	Milk	Oils
Goal Amount						
Estimate Your Total						
Increase ⬆ or Decrease ⬇ ?						

PHYSICAL ACTIVITY

Description: _____

Steps/Miles/Minutes: _____

SPIRITUAL ACTIVITY

Description: _____

_____

Live It Tracker

Name: _____ My week at a glance: ☐ Great ☐ So-so ☐ Not so great

Date: _____ Week #: _____ Calorie Range: _____ My food goal for next week: _____

Activity Level: None, < 30 min/day, 30-60 min/day, 60+ min/day   My activity goal for next week: _____

Scripture Memory Verse: _____

RECOMMENDED DAILY AMOUNT OF FOOD FROM EACH GROUP

Group	Daily Calories							
	1300-1400	1500-1600	1700-1800	1900-2000	2100-2200	2300-2400	2500-2600	2700-2800
Fruits	1.5-2 c.	1.5-2 c.	1.5-2 c.	2-2.5 c.	2-2.5 c.	2.5-3.5 c.	3.5-4.5 c.	3.5-4.5 c.
Vegetables	1.5-2 c.	2-2.5 c.	2.5-3 c.	2.5-3 c.	3-3.5 c.	3.5-4.5 c.	4.5-5 c.	4.5-5 c.
Grains	5 oz-eq.	5-6 oz-eq.	6-7 oz-eq.	6-7 oz-eq.	7-8 oz-eq.	8-9 oz-eq.	9-10 oz-eq.	10-11 oz-eq.
Meat & Beans	4 oz-eq.	5 oz-eq.	5-5.5 oz-eq.	5.5-6.5 oz-eq.	6.5-7 oz-eq.	7-7.5 oz-eq.	7-7.5 oz-eq.	7.5-8 oz-eq.
Milk	2-3 c.	3 c.	3 c.	3 c.	3 c.	3 c.	3 c.	3 c.
Healthy Oils	4 tsp.	5 tsp.	5 tsp.	6 tsp.	6 tsp.	7 tsp.	8 tsp.	8 tsp.

Day One

FOOD CHOICES

Breakfast: _____ Lunch: _____

Dinner: _____ Snacks: _____

Group	Fruits	Vegetables	Grains	Meat & Beans	Milk	Oils
Goal Amount						
Estimate Your Total						
Increase ⬆ or Decrease ⬇ ?						

PHYSICAL ACTIVITY   **SPIRITUAL ACTIVITY**

Description: _____ Description: _____

Steps/Miles/Minutes: _____

Day Two

FOOD CHOICES

Breakfast: _____ Lunch: _____

Dinner: _____ Snacks: _____

Group	Fruits	Vegetables	Grains	Meat & Beans	Milk	Oils
Goal Amount						
Estimate Your Total						
Increase ⬆ or Decrease ⬇ ?						

PHYSICAL ACTIVITY   **SPIRITUAL ACTIVITY**

Description: _____ Description: _____

Steps/Miles/Minutes: _____

Day Three

FOOD CHOICES

Breakfast: _____ Lunch: _____

Dinner: _____ Snacks: _____

Group	Fruits	Vegetables	Grains	Meat & Beans	Milk	Oils
Goal Amount						
Estimate Your Total						
Increase ⬆ or Decrease ⬇ ?						

PHYSICAL ACTIVITY   **SPIRITUAL ACTIVITY**

Description: _____ Description: _____

Steps/Miles/Minutes: _____

Day Four

FOOD CHOICES

Breakfast: _____ Lunch: _____

Dinner: _____ Snacks: _____

Group	Fruits	Vegetables	Grains	Meat & Beans	Milk	Oils
Goal Amount						
Estimate Your Total						
Increase ⇧ or Decrease ⇩ ?						

PHYSICAL ACTIVITY

Description: _____

Steps/Miles/Minutes: _____

SPIRITUAL ACTIVITY

Description: _____

_____

Day Five

FOOD CHOICES

Breakfast: _____ Lunch: _____

Dinner: _____ Snacks: _____

Group	Fruits	Vegetables	Grains	Meat & Beans	Milk	Oils
Goal Amount						
Estimate Your Total						
Increase ⇧ or Decrease ⇩ ?						

PHYSICAL ACTIVITY

Description: _____

Steps/Miles/Minutes: _____

SPIRITUAL ACTIVITY

Description: _____

_____

Day Six

FOOD CHOICES

Breakfast: _____ Lunch: _____

Dinner: _____ Snacks: _____

Group	Fruits	Vegetables	Grains	Meat & Beans	Milk	Oils
Goal Amount						
Estimate Your Total						
Increase ⇧ or Decrease ⇩ ?						

PHYSICAL ACTIVITY

Description: _____

Steps/Miles/Minutes: _____

SPIRITUAL ACTIVITY

Description: _____

_____

Day Seven

FOOD CHOICES

Breakfast: _____ Lunch: _____

Dinner: _____ Snacks: _____

Group	Fruits	Vegetables	Grains	Meat & Beans	Milk	Oils
Goal Amount						
Estimate Your Total						
Increase ⇧ or Decrease ⇩ ?						

PHYSICAL ACTIVITY

Description: _____

Steps/Miles/Minutes: _____

SPIRITUAL ACTIVITY

Description: _____

_____

Live It Tracker

Name: _____   My week at a glance: ☐ Great ☐ So-so ☐ Not so great

Date: _____ Week #: _____ Calorie Range: _____   My food goal for next week: _____

Activity Level: None, < 30 min/day, 30-60 min/day, 60+ min/day   My activity goal for next week: _____

Scripture Memory Verse: _____

RECOMMENDED DAILY AMOUNT OF FOOD FROM EACH GROUP

Group	Daily Calories							
	1300-1400	1500-1600	1700-1800	1900-2000	2100-2200	2300-2400	2500-2600	2700-2800
Fruits	1.5-2 c.	1.5-2 c.	1.5-2 c.	2-2.5 c.	2-2.5 c.	2.5-3.5 c.	3.5-4.5 c.	3.5-4.5 c.
Vegetables	1.5-2 c.	2-2.5 c.	2.5-3 c.	2.5-3 c.	3-3.5 c.	3.5-4.5 c.	4.5-5 c.	4.5-5 c.
Grains	5 oz-eq.	5-6 oz-eq.	6-7 oz-eq.	6-7 oz-eq.	7-8 oz-eq.	8-9 oz-eq.	9-10 oz-eq.	10-11 oz-eq.
Meat & Beans	4 oz-eq.	5 oz-eq.	5-5.5 oz-eq.	5.5-6.5 oz-eq.	6.5-7 oz-eq.	7-7.5 oz-eq.	7-7.5 oz-eq.	7.5-8 oz-eq.
Milk	2-3 c.	3 c.	3 c.	3 c.	3 c.	3 c.	3 c.	3 c.
Healthy Oils	4 tsp.	5 tsp.	5 tsp.	6 tsp.	6 tsp.	7 tsp.	8 tsp.	8 tsp.

Day One

FOOD CHOICES

Breakfast: _____   Lunch: _____

Dinner: _____   Snacks: _____

Group	Fruits	Vegetables	Grains	Meat & Beans	Milk	Oils
Goal Amount						
Estimate Your Total						
Increase ⇧ or Decrease ⇩ ?						

PHYSICAL ACTIVITY   **SPIRITUAL ACTIVITY**

Description: _____   Description: _____

Steps/Miles/Minutes: _____

Day Two

FOOD CHOICES

Breakfast: _____   Lunch: _____

Dinner: _____   Snacks: _____

Group	Fruits	Vegetables	Grains	Meat & Beans	Milk	Oils
Goal Amount						
Estimate Your Total						
Increase ⇧ or Decrease ⇩ ?						

PHYSICAL ACTIVITY   **SPIRITUAL ACTIVITY**

Description: _____   Description: _____

Steps/Miles/Minutes: _____

Day Three

FOOD CHOICES

Breakfast: _____   Lunch: _____

Dinner: _____   Snacks: _____

Group	Fruits	Vegetables	Grains	Meat & Beans	Milk	Oils
Goal Amount						
Estimate Your Total						
Increase ⇧ or Decrease ⇩ ?						

PHYSICAL ACTIVITY   **SPIRITUAL ACTIVITY**

Description: _____   Description: _____

Steps/Miles/Minutes: _____

FOOD CHOICES

Day Four

Breakfast: _____   Lunch: _____

Dinner: _____   Snacks: _____

Group	Fruits	Vegetables	Grains	Meat & Beans	Milk	Oils
Goal Amount						
Estimate Your Total						
Increase ⇧ or Decrease ⇩ ?						

PHYSICAL ACTIVITY

Description: _____

Steps/Miles/Minutes: _____

SPIRITUAL ACTIVITY

Description: _____

_____

FOOD CHOICES

Day Five

Breakfast: _____   Lunch: _____

Dinner: _____   Snacks: _____

Group	Fruits	Vegetables	Grains	Meat & Beans	Milk	Oils
Goal Amount						
Estimate Your Total						
Increase ⇧ or Decrease ⇩ ?						

PHYSICAL ACTIVITY

Description: _____

Steps/Miles/Minutes: _____

SPIRITUAL ACTIVITY

Description: _____

_____

FOOD CHOICES

Day Six

Breakfast: _____   Lunch: _____

Dinner: _____   Snacks: _____

Group	Fruits	Vegetables	Grains	Meat & Beans	Milk	Oils
Goal Amount						
Estimate Your Total						
Increase ⇧ or Decrease ⇩ ?						

PHYSICAL ACTIVITY

Description: _____

Steps/Miles/Minutes: _____

SPIRITUAL ACTIVITY

Description: _____

_____

FOOD CHOICES

Day Seven

Breakfast: _____   Lunch: _____

Dinner: _____   Snacks: _____

Group	Fruits	Vegetables	Grains	Meat & Beans	Milk	Oils
Goal Amount						
Estimate Your Total						
Increase ⇧ or Decrease ⇩ ?						

PHYSICAL ACTIVITY

Description: _____

Steps/Miles/Minutes: _____

SPIRITUAL ACTIVITY

Description: _____

_____

Live It Tracker

Name: _____   My week at a glance: ❏ Great ❏ So-so ❏ Not so great

Date: _____ Week #: _____ Calorie Range: _____   My food goal for next week: _____

Activity Level: None, < 30 min/day, 30-60 min/day, 60+ min/day   My activity goal for next week: _____

Scripture Memory Verse: _____

RECOMMENDED DAILY AMOUNT OF FOOD FROM EACH GROUP

Group	Daily Calories							
	1300-1400	1500-1600	1700-1800	1900-2000	2100-2200	2300-2400	2500-2600	2700-2800
Fruits	1.5-2 c.	1.5-2 c.	1.5-2 c.	2-2.5 c.	2-2.5 c.	2.5-3.5 c.	3.5-4.5 c.	3.5-4.5 c.
Vegetables	1.5-2 c.	2-2.5 c.	2.5-3 c.	2.5-3 c.	3-3.5 c.	3.5-4.5 c.	4.5-5 c.	4.5-5 c.
Grains	5 oz-eq.	5-6 oz-eq.	6-7 oz-eq.	6-7 oz-eq.	7-8 oz-eq.	8-9 oz-eq.	9-10 oz-eq.	10-11 oz-eq.
Meat & Beans	4 oz-eq.	5 oz-eq.	5-5.5 oz-eq.	5.5-6.5 oz eq.	6.5-7 oz-eq.	7-7.5 oz-eq.	7-7.5 oz-eq.	7.5-8 oz-eq.
Milk	2-3 c.	3 c.	3 c.	3 c.	3 c.	3 c.	3 c.	3 c.
Healthy Oils	4 tsp.	5 tsp.	5 tsp.	6 tsp.	6 tsp.	7 tsp.	8 tsp.	8 tsp.

Day One

FOOD CHOICES
Breakfast: _____   Lunch: _____
Dinner: _____   Snacks: _____

Group	Fruits	Vegetables	Grains	Meat & Beans	Milk	Oils
Goal Amount						
Estimate Your Total						
Increase ⇧ or Decrease ⇩ ?						

PHYSICAL ACTIVITY
Description: _____
Steps/Miles/Minutes: _____

SPIRITUAL ACTIVITY
Description: _____

Day Two

FOOD CHOICES
Breakfast: _____   Lunch: _____
Dinner: _____   Snacks: _____

Group	Fruits	Vegetables	Grains	Meat & Beans	Milk	Oils
Goal Amount						
Estimate Your Total						
Increase ⇧ or Decrease ⇩ ?						

PHYSICAL ACTIVITY
Description: _____
Steps/Miles/Minutes: _____

SPIRITUAL ACTIVITY
Description: _____

Day Three

FOOD CHOICES
Breakfast: _____   Lunch: _____
Dinner: _____   Snacks: _____

Group	Fruits	Vegetables	Grains	Meat & Beans	Milk	Oils
Goal Amount						
Estimate Your Total						
Increase ⇧ or Decrease ⇩ ?						

PHYSICAL ACTIVITY
Description: _____
Steps/Miles/Minutes: _____

SPIRITUAL ACTIVITY
Description: _____

Day Four

FOOD CHOICES

Breakfast: _____ Lunch: _____

Dinner: _____ Snacks: _____

Group	Fruits	Vegetables	Grains	Meat & Beans	Milk	Oils
Goal Amount						
Estimate Your Total						
Increase ⇧ or Decrease ⇩ ?						

PHYSICAL ACTIVITY

Description: _____

Steps/Miles/Minutes: _____

SPIRITUAL ACTIVITY

Description: _____

_____

Day Five

FOOD CHOICES

Breakfast: _____ Lunch: _____

Dinner: _____ Snacks: _____

Group	Fruits	Vegetables	Grains	Meat & Beans	Milk	Oils
Goal Amount						
Estimate Your Total						
Increase ⇧ or Decrease ⇩ ?						

PHYSICAL ACTIVITY

Description: _____

Steps/Miles/Minutes: _____

SPIRITUAL ACTIVITY

Description: _____

_____

Day Six

FOOD CHOICES

Breakfast: _____ Lunch: _____

Dinner: _____ Snacks: _____

Group	Fruits	Vegetables	Grains	Meat & Beans	Milk	Oils
Goal Amount						
Estimate Your Total						
Increase ⇧ or Decrease ⇩ ?						

PHYSICAL ACTIVITY

Description: _____

Steps/Miles/Minutes: _____

SPIRITUAL ACTIVITY

Description: _____

_____

Day Seven

FOOD CHOICES

Breakfast: _____ Lunch: _____

Dinner: _____ Snacks: _____

Group	Fruits	Vegetables	Grains	Meat & Beans	Milk	Oils
Goal Amount						
Estimate Your Total						
Increase ⇧ or Decrease ⇩ ?						

PHYSICAL ACTIVITY

Description: _____

Steps/Miles/Minutes: _____

SPIRITUAL ACTIVITY

Description: _____

_____

Live It Tracker

Name: _____ My week at a glance: ☐ Great ☐ So-so ☐ Not so great

Date: _____ Week #: _____ Calorie Range: _____ My food goal for next week: _____

Activity Level: None, < 30 min/day, 30-60 min/day, 60+ min/day   My activity goal for next week: _____

Scripture Memory Verse: _____

RECOMMENDED DAILY AMOUNT OF FOOD FROM EACH GROUP

Group	Daily Calories							
	1300-1400	1500-1600	1700-1800	1900-2000	2100-2200	2300-2400	2500-2600	2700-2800
Fruits	1.5-2 c.	1.5-2 c.	1.5-2 c.	2-2.5 c.	2-2.5 c.	2.5-3.5 c.	3.5-4.5 c.	3.5-4.5 c.
Vegetables	1.5-2 c.	2-2.5 c.	2.5-3 c.	2.5-3 c.	3-3.5 c.	3.5-4.5 c.	4.5-5 c.	4.5-5 c.
Grains	5 oz-eq.	5-6 oz-eq.	6-7 oz-eq.	6-7 oz-eq.	7-8 oz-eq.	8-9 oz-eq.	9-10 oz-eq.	10-11 oz-eq.
Meat & Beans	4 oz-eq.	5 oz-eq.	5-5.5 oz-eq.	5.5-6.5 oz-eq.	6.5-7 oz-eq.	7-7.5 oz-eq.	7-7.5 oz-eq.	7.5-8 oz-eq.
Milk	2-3 c.	3 c.	3 c.	3 c.	3 c.	3 c.	3 c.	3 c.
Healthy Oils	4 tsp.	5 tsp.	5 tsp.	6 tsp.	6 tsp.	7 tsp.	8 tsp.	8 tsp.

FOOD CHOICES
Breakfast: _____ Lunch: _____

Dinner: _____ Snacks: _____

Day One

Group	Fruits	Vegetables	Grains	Meat & Beans	Milk	Oils
Goal Amount						
Estimate Your Total						
Increase ⬆ or Decrease ⬇ ?						

PHYSICAL ACTIVITY
Description: _____

Steps/Miles/Minutes: _____

SPIRITUAL ACTIVITY
Description: _____

_____

FOOD CHOICES
Breakfast: _____ Lunch: _____

Dinner: _____ Snacks: _____

Day Two

Group	Fruits	Vegetables	Grains	Meat & Beans	Milk	Oils
Goal Amount						
Estimate Your Total						
Increase ⬆ or Decrease ⬇ ?						

PHYSICAL ACTIVITY
Description: _____

Steps/Miles/Minutes: _____

SPIRITUAL ACTIVITY
Description: _____

_____

FOOD CHOICES
Breakfast: _____ Lunch: _____

Dinner: _____ Snacks: _____

Day Three

Group	Fruits	Vegetables	Grains	Meat & Beans	Milk	Oils
Goal Amount						
Estimate Your Total						
Increase ⬆ or Decrease ⬇ ?						

PHYSICAL ACTIVITY
Description: _____

Steps/Miles/Minutes: _____

SPIRITUAL ACTIVITY
Description: _____

_____

Day Four

FOOD CHOICES
Breakfast: _____ Lunch: _____
Dinner: _____ Snacks: _____

Group	Fruits	Vegetables	Grains	Meat & Beans	Milk	Oils
Goal Amount						
Estimate Your Total						
Increase ⇧ or Decrease ⇩ ?						

PHYSICAL ACTIVITY
Description: _____
Steps/Miles/Minutes: _____

SPIRITUAL ACTIVITY
Description: _____
_____

Day Five

FOOD CHOICES
Breakfast: _____ Lunch: _____
Dinner: _____ Snacks: _____

Group	Fruits	Vegetables	Grains	Meat & Beans	Milk	Oils
Goal Amount						
Estimate Your Total						
Increase ⇧ or Decrease ⇩ ?						

PHYSICAL ACTIVITY
Description: _____
Steps/Miles/Minutes: _____

SPIRITUAL ACTIVITY
Description: _____
_____

Day Six

FOOD CHOICES
Breakfast: _____ Lunch: _____
Dinner: _____ Snacks: _____

Group	Fruits	Vegetables	Grains	Meat & Beans	Milk	Oils
Goal Amount						
Estimate Your Total						
Increase ⇧ or Decrease ⇩ ?						

PHYSICAL ACTIVITY
Description: _____
Steps/Miles/Minutes: _____

SPIRITUAL ACTIVITY
Description: _____
_____

Day Seven

FOOD CHOICES
Breakfast: _____ Lunch: _____
Dinner: _____ Snacks: _____

Group	Fruits	Vegetables	Grains	Meat & Beans	Milk	Oils
Goal Amount						
Estimate Your Total						
Increase ⇧ or Decrease ⇩ ?						

PHYSICAL ACTIVITY
Description: _____
Steps/Miles/Minutes: _____

SPIRITUAL ACTIVITY
Description: _____
_____

Live It Tracker

Name: _____ My week at a glance: ☐ Great ☐ So-so ☐ Not so great

Date: _____ Week #: _____ Calorie Range: _____ My food goal for next week: _____

Activity Level: None, < 30 min/day, 30-60 min/day, 60+ min/day   My activity goal for next week: _____

Scripture Memory Verse: _____

RECOMMENDED DAILY AMOUNT OF FOOD FROM EACH GROUP

Group	Daily Calories							
	1300-1400	1500-1600	1700-1800	1900-2000	2100-2200	2300-2400	2500-2600	2700-2800
Fruits	1.5-2 c.	1.5-2 c.	1.5-2 c.	2-2.5 c.	2-2.5 c.	2.5-3.5 c.	3.5-4.5 c.	3.5-4.5 c.
Vegetables	1.5-2 c.	2-2.5 c.	2.5-3 c.	2.5-3 c.	3-3.5 c.	3.5-4.5 c.	4.5-5 c.	4.5-5 c.
Grains	5 oz-eq.	5-6 oz-eq.	6-7 oz-eq.	6-7 oz-eq.	7-8 oz-eq.	8-9 oz-eq.	9-10 oz-eq.	10-11 oz-eq.
Meat & Beans	4 oz-eq.	5 oz-eq.	5 5.5 oz-eq.	5.5-6.5 oz-eq.	6.5-7 oz-eq.	7-7.5 oz-eq.	7-7.5 oz-eq.	7.5-8 oz-eq.
Milk	2.3 c.	3 c.	3 c.	3 c.	3 c.	3 c.	3 c.	3 c.
Healthy Oils	4 tsp.	5 tsp.	5 tsp.	6 tsp.	6 tsp.	7 tsp.	8 tsp.	8 tsp.

FOOD CHOICES

Breakfast: _____ Lunch: _____

Dinner: _____ Snacks: _____

Day One

Group	Fruits	Vegetables	Grains	Meat & Beans	Milk	Oils
Goal Amount						
Estimate Your Total						
Increase ⇧ or Decrease ⇩ ?						

PHYSICAL ACTIVITY

Description: _____

Steps/Miles/Minutes: _____

SPIRITUAL ACTIVITY

Description: _____

FOOD CHOICES

Breakfast: _____ Lunch: _____

Dinner: _____ Snacks: _____

Day Two

Group	Fruits	Vegetables	Grains	Meat & Beans	Milk	Oils
Goal Amount						
Estimate Your Total						
Increase ⇧ or Decrease ⇩ ?						

PHYSICAL ACTIVITY

Description: _____

Steps/Miles/Minutes: _____

SPIRITUAL ACTIVITY

Description: _____

FOOD CHOICES

Breakfast: _____ Lunch: _____

Dinner: _____ Snacks: _____

Day Three

Group	Fruits	Vegetables	Grains	Meat & Beans	Milk	Oils
Goal Amount						
Estimate Your Total						
Increase ⇧ or Decrease ⇩ ?						

PHYSICAL ACTIVITY

Description: _____

Steps/Miles/Minutes: _____

SPIRITUAL ACTIVITY

Description: _____

Day Four

FOOD CHOICES

Breakfast: _____ Lunch: _____

Dinner: _____ Snacks: _____

Group	Fruits	Vegetables	Grains	Meat & Beans	Milk	Oils
Goal Amount						
Estimate Your Total						
Increase ⇧ or Decrease ⇩ ?						

PHYSICAL ACTIVITY

Description: _____

Steps/Miles/Minutes: _____

SPIRITUAL ACTIVITY

Description: _____

_____

Day Five

FOOD CHOICES

Breakfast: _____ Lunch: _____

Dinner: _____ Snacks: _____

Group	Fruits	Vegetables	Grains	Meat & Beans	Milk	Oils
Goal Amount						
Estimate Your Total						
Increase ⇧ or Decrease ⇩ ?						

PHYSICAL ACTIVITY

Description: _____

Steps/Miles/Minutes: _____

SPIRITUAL ACTIVITY

Description: _____

_____

Day Six

FOOD CHOICES

Breakfast: _____ Lunch: _____

Dinner: _____ Snacks: _____

Group	Fruits	Vegetables	Grains	Meat & Beans	Milk	Oils
Goal Amount						
Estimate Your Total						
Increase ⇧ or Decrease ⇩ ?						

PHYSICAL ACTIVITY

Description: _____

Steps/Miles/Minutes: _____

SPIRITUAL ACTIVITY

Description: _____

_____

Day Seven

FOOD CHOICES

Breakfast: _____ Lunch: _____

Dinner: _____ Snacks: _____

Group	Fruits	Vegetables	Grains	Meat & Beans	Milk	Oils
Goal Amount						
Estimate Your Total						
Increase ⇧ or Decrease ⇩ ?						

PHYSICAL ACTIVITY

Description: _____

Steps/Miles/Minutes: _____

SPIRITUAL ACTIVITY

Description: _____

_____

Live It Tracker

RECOMMENDED DAILY AMOUNT OF FOOD FROM EACH GROUP

Group	Daily Calories							
	1300-1400	1500-1600	1700-1800	1900-2000	2100-2200	2300-2400	2500-2600	2700-2800
Fruits	1.5-2 c.	1.5-2 c.	1.5-2 c.	2-2.5 c.	2-2.5 c.	2.5-3.5 c.	3.5-4.5 c.	3.5-4.5 c.
Vegetables	1.5-2 c.	2-2.5 c.	2.5-3 c.	2.5-3 c.	3-3.5 c.	3.5-4.5 c.	4.5-5 c.	4.5-5 c.
Grains	5 oz-eq.	5-6 oz-eq.	6-7 oz-eq.	6-7 oz-eq.	7-8 oz-eq.	8-9 oz-eq.	9-10 oz-eq.	10-11 oz-eq.
Meat & Beans	4 oz-eq.	5 oz-eq.	5-5.5 oz eq.	5.5-6.5 oz-eq.	6.5-7 oz-eq.	7-7.5 oz-eq.	7-7.5 oz-eq.	7.5-8 oz-eq.
Milk	2-3 c.	3 c.	3 c.	3 c.	3 c.	3 c.	3 c.	3 c.
Healthy Oils	4 tsp.	5 tsp.	5 tsp.	6 tsp.	6 tsp.	7 tsp.	8 tsp.	8 tsp.

Day One

FOOD CHOICES
Breakfast: _____   Lunch: _____

Dinner: _____   Snacks: _____

Group	Fruits	Vegetables	Grains	Meat & Beans	Milk	Oils
Goal Amount						
Estimate Your Total						
Increase ⇧ or Decrease ⇩ ?						

PHYSICAL ACTIVITY
Description: _____

Steps/Miles/Minutes: _____

SPIRITUAL ACTIVITY
Description: _____

Day Two

FOOD CHOICES
Breakfast: _____   Lunch: _____

Dinner: _____   Snacks: _____

Group	Fruits	Vegetables	Grains	Meat & Beans	Milk	Oils
Goal Amount						
Estimate Your Total						
Increase ⇧ or Decrease ⇩ ?						

PHYSICAL ACTIVITY
Description: _____

Steps/Miles/Minutes: _____

SPIRITUAL ACTIVITY
Description: _____

Day Three

FOOD CHOICES
Breakfast: _____   Lunch: _____

Dinner: _____   Snacks: _____

Group	Fruits	Vegetables	Grains	Meat & Beans	Milk	Oils
Goal Amount						
Estimate Your Total						
Increase ⇧ or Decrease ⇩ ?						

PHYSICAL ACTIVITY
Description: _____

Steps/Miles/Minutes: _____

SPIRITUAL ACTIVITY
Description: _____

Day Four

FOOD CHOICES

Breakfast: _____ Lunch: _____

Dinner: _____ Snacks: _____

Group	Fruits	Vegetables	Grains	Meat & Beans	Milk	Oils
Goal Amount						
Estimate Your Total						
Increase ⇧ or Decrease ⇩ ?						

PHYSICAL ACTIVITY

Description: _____

Steps/Miles/Minutes: _____

SPIRITUAL ACTIVITY

Description: _____

_____

Day Five

FOOD CHOICES

Breakfast: _____ Lunch: _____

Dinner: _____ Snacks: _____

Group	Fruits	Vegetables	Grains	Meat & Beans	Milk	Oils
Goal Amount						
Estimate Your Total						
Increase ⇧ or Decrease ⇩ ?						

PHYSICAL ACTIVITY

Description: _____

Steps/Miles/Minutes: _____

SPIRITUAL ACTIVITY

Description: _____

_____

Day Six

FOOD CHOICES

Breakfast: _____ Lunch: _____

Dinner: _____ Snacks: _____

Group	Fruits	Vegetables	Grains	Meat & Beans	Milk	Oils
Goal Amount						
Estimate Your Total						
Increase ⇧ or Decrease ⇩ ?						

PHYSICAL ACTIVITY

Description: _____

Steps/Miles/Minutes: _____

SPIRITUAL ACTIVITY

Description: _____

_____

Day Seven

FOOD CHOICES

Breakfast: _____ Lunch: _____

Dinner: _____ Snacks: _____

Group	Fruits	Vegetables	Grains	Meat & Beans	Milk	Oils
Goal Amount						
Estimate Your Total						
Increase ⇧ or Decrease ⇩ ?						

PHYSICAL ACTIVITY

Description: _____

Steps/Miles/Minutes: _____

SPIRITUAL ACTIVITY

Description: _____

_____

Live It Tracker

Name: _____   My week at a glance: ☐ Great ☐ So-so ☐ Not so great

Date: _____ Week #: _____ Calorie Range: _____   My food goal for next week: _____

Activity Level: None, < 30 min/day, 30-60 min/day, 60+ min/day   My activity goal for next week: _____

Scripture Memory Verse: _____

RECOMMENDED DAILY AMOUNT OF FOOD FROM EACH GROUP

Group	Daily Calories							
	1300-1400	1500-1600	1700-1800	1900-2000	2100-2200	2300-2400	2500-2600	2700-2800
Fruits	1.5-2 c.	1.5-2 c.	1.5-2 c.	2-2.5 c.	2-2.5 c.	2.5-3.5 c.	3.5-4.5 c.	3.5-4.5 c.
Vegetables	1.5-2 c.	2-2.5 c.	2.5-3 c.	2.5-3 c.	3-3.5 c.	3.5-4.5 c.	4.5-5 c.	4.5-5 c.
Grains	5 oz-eq.	5-6 oz-eq.	6-7 oz-eq.	6-7 oz-eq.	7-8 oz-eq.	8-9 oz-eq.	9-10 oz-eq.	10-11 oz-eq.
Meat & Beans	4 oz-eq.	5 oz-eq.	5-5.5 oz eq.	5.5-6.5 oz-eq.	6.5-7 oz-eq.	7-7.5 oz-eq.	7-7.5 oz-eq.	7.5-8 oz-eq.
Milk	2-3 c.	3 c.	3 c.	3 c.	3 c.	3 c.	3 c.	3 c.
Healthy Oils	4 tsp.	5 tsp.	5 tsp.	6 tsp.	6 tsp.	7 tsp.	8 tsp.	8 tsp.

Day One

FOOD CHOICES
Breakfast: _____   Lunch: _____

Dinner: _____   Snacks: _____

Group	Fruits	Vegetables	Grains	Meat & Beans	Milk	Oils
Goal Amount						
Estimate Your Total						
Increase ⇧ or Decrease ⇩ ?						

PHYSICAL ACTIVITY   SPIRITUAL ACTIVITY

Description: _____   Description: _____

Steps/Miles/Minutes: _____

Day Two

FOOD CHOICES
Breakfast: _____   Lunch: _____

Dinner: _____   Snacks: _____

Group	Fruits	Vegetables	Grains	Meat & Beans	Milk	Oils
Goal Amount						
Estimate Your Total						
Increase ⇧ or Decrease ⇩ ?						

PHYSICAL ACTIVITY   SPIRITUAL ACTIVITY

Description: _____   Description: _____

Steps/Miles/Minutes: _____

Day Three

FOOD CHOICES
Breakfast: _____   Lunch: _____

Dinner: _____   Snacks: _____

Group	Fruits	Vegetables	Grains	Meat & Beans	Milk	Oils
Goal Amount						
Estimate Your Total						
Increase ⇧ or Decrease ⇩ ?						

PHYSICAL ACTIVITY   SPIRITUAL ACTIVITY

Description: _____   Description: _____

Steps/Miles/Minutes: _____

Day Four

FOOD CHOICES

Breakfast: _____ Lunch: _____

Dinner: _____ Snacks: _____

Group	Fruits	Vegetables	Grains	Meat & Beans	Milk	Oils
Goal Amount						
Estimate Your Total						
Increase ⇧ or Decrease ⇩ ?						

PHYSICAL ACTIVITY

Description: _____

Steps/Miles/Minutes: _____

SPIRITUAL ACTIVITY

Description: _____

_____

Day Five

FOOD CHOICES

Breakfast: _____ Lunch: _____

Dinner: _____ Snacks: _____

Group	Fruits	Vegetables	Grains	Meat & Beans	Milk	Oils
Goal Amount						
Estimate Your Total						
Increase ⇧ or Decrease ⇩ ?						

PHYSICAL ACTIVITY

Description: _____

Steps/Miles/Minutes: _____

SPIRITUAL ACTIVITY

Description: _____

_____

Day Six

FOOD CHOICES

Breakfast: _____ Lunch: _____

Dinner: _____ Snacks: _____

Group	Fruits	Vegetables	Grains	Meat & Beans	Milk	Oils
Goal Amount						
Estimate Your Total						
Increase ⇧ or Decrease ⇩ ?						

PHYSICAL ACTIVITY

Description: _____

Steps/Miles/Minutes: _____

SPIRITUAL ACTIVITY

Description: _____

_____

Day Seven

FOOD CHOICES

Breakfast: _____ Lunch: _____

Dinner: _____ Snacks: _____

Group	Fruits	Vegetables	Grains	Meat & Beans	Milk	Oils
Goal Amount						
Estimate Your Total						
Increase ⇧ or Decrease ⇩ ?						

PHYSICAL ACTIVITY

Description: _____

Steps/Miles/Minutes: _____

SPIRITUAL ACTIVITY

Description: _____

_____

Live It Tracker

Name: _____   My week at a glance: ❑ Great ❑ So-so ❑ Not so great

Date: _____ Week #: _____ Calorie Range: _____   My food goal for next week: _____

Activity Level: None, < 30 min/day, 30-60 min/day, 60+ min/day   My activity goal for next week: _____

Scripture Memory Verse: _____

_____

RECOMMENDED DAILY AMOUNT OF FOOD FROM EACH GROUP

Group	Daily Calories							
	1300-1400	1500-1600	1700-1800	1900-2000	2100-2200	2300-2400	2500-2600	2700-2800
Fruits	1.5-2 c.	1.5-2 c.	1.5-2 c.	2-2.5 c.	2-2.5 c.	2.5-3.5 c.	3.5-4.5 c.	3.5-4.5 c.
Vegetables	1.5-2 c.	2-2.5 c.	2.5-3 c.	2.5-3 c.	3-3.5 c.	3.5-4.5 c.	4.5-5 c.	4.5-5 c.
Grains	5 oz-eq.	5-6 oz-eq.	6-7 oz-eq.	6-7 oz-eq.	7-8 oz-eq.	8-9 oz-eq.	9-10 oz-eq.	10-11 oz-eq.
Meat & Beans	4 oz-eq.	5 oz-eq.	5-5.5 oz-eq.	5.5-6.5 oz-eq.	6.5-7 oz-eq.	7-7.5 oz-eq.	7-7.5 oz-eq.	7.5-8 oz-eq.
Milk	2-3 c.	3 c.	3 c.	3 c.	3 c.	3 c.	3 c.	3 c.
Healthy Oils	4 tsp.	5 tsp.	5 tsp.	6 tsp.	6 tsp.	7 tsp.	8 tsp.	8 tsp.

Day One

FOOD CHOICES

Breakfast: _____   Lunch: _____

Dinner: _____   Snacks: _____

Group	Fruits	Vegetables	Grains	Meat & Beans	Milk	Oils
Goal Amount						
Estimate Your Total						
Increase ⇧ or Decrease ⇩ ?						

PHYSICAL ACTIVITY

Description: _____

Steps/Miles/Minutes: _____

SPIRITUAL ACTIVITY

Description: _____

Day Two

FOOD CHOICES

Breakfast: _____   Lunch: _____

Dinner: _____   Snacks: _____

Group	Fruits	Vegetables	Grains	Meat & Beans	Milk	Oils
Goal Amount						
Estimate Your Total						
Increase ⇧ or Decrease ⇩ ?						

PHYSICAL ACTIVITY

Description: _____

Steps/Miles/Minutes: _____

SPIRITUAL ACTIVITY

Description: _____

Day Three

FOOD CHOICES

Breakfast: _____   Lunch: _____

Dinner: _____   Snacks: _____

Group	Fruits	Vegetables	Grains	Meat & Beans	Milk	Oils
Goal Amount						
Estimate Your Total						
Increase ⇧ or Decrease ⇩ ?						

PHYSICAL ACTIVITY

Description: _____

Steps/Miles/Minutes: _____

SPIRITUAL ACTIVITY

Description: _____

Day Four

FOOD CHOICES

Breakfast: _____   Lunch: _____

Dinner: _____   Snacks: _____

Group	Fruits	Vegetables	Grains	Meat & Beans	Milk	Oils
Goal Amount						
Estimate Your Total						
Increase ⇧ or Decrease ⇩ ?						

PHYSICAL ACTIVITY   **SPIRITUAL ACTIVITY**

Description: _____   Description: _____

Steps/Miles/Minutes: _____   _____

Day Five

FOOD CHOICES

Breakfast: _____   Lunch: _____

Dinner: _____   Snacks: _____

Group	Fruits	Vegetables	Grains	Meat & Beans	Milk	Oils
Goal Amount						
Estimate Your Total						
Increase ⇧ or Decrease ⇩ ?						

PHYSICAL ACTIVITY   **SPIRITUAL ACTIVITY**

Description: _____   Description: _____

Steps/Miles/Minutes: _____   _____

Day Six

FOOD CHOICES

Breakfast: _____   Lunch: _____

Dinner: _____   Snacks: _____

Group	Fruits	Vegetables	Grains	Meat & Beans	Milk	Oils
Goal Amount						
Estimate Your Total						
Increase ⇧ or Decrease ⇩ ?						

PHYSICAL ACTIVITY   **SPIRITUAL ACTIVITY**

Description: _____   Description: _____

Steps/Miles/Minutes: _____   _____

Day Seven

FOOD CHOICES

Breakfast: _____   Lunch: _____

Dinner: _____   Snacks: _____

Group	Fruits	Vegetables	Grains	Meat & Beans	Milk	Oils
Goal Amount						
Estimate Your Total						
Increase ⇧ or Decrease ⇩ ?						

PHYSICAL ACTIVITY   **SPIRITUAL ACTIVITY**

Description: _____   Description: _____

Steps/Miles/Minutes: _____   _____

Live It Tracker

Name: _____ My week at a glance: ☐ Great ☐ So-so ☐ Not so great

Date: _____ Week #: _____ Calorie Range: _____ My food goal for next week: _____

Activity Level: None, < 30 min/day, 30-60 min/day, 60+ min/day   My activity goal for next week: _____

Scripture Memory Verse: _____
_____

RECOMMENDED DAILY AMOUNT OF FOOD FROM EACH GROUP

Group	Daily Calories							
	1300-1400	1500-1600	1700-1800	1900-2000	2100-2200	2300-2400	2500-2600	2700-2800
Fruits	1.5-2 c.	1.5-2 c.	1.5-2 c.	2-2.5 c.	2-2.5 c.	2.5-3.5 c.	3.5-4.5 c.	3.5-4.5 c.
Vegetables	1.5-2 c.	2-2.5 c.	2.5-3 c.	2.5-3 c.	3-3.5 c.	3.5-4.5 c.	4.5-5 c.	4.5-5 c.
Grains	5 oz-eq.	5-6 oz-eq.	6-7 oz-eq.	6-7 oz-eq.	7-8 oz-eq.	8-9 oz-eq.	9-10 oz-eq.	10-11 oz-eq.
Meat & Beans	4 oz-eq.	5 oz-eq.	5-5.5 oz-eq.	5.5-6.5 oz-eq.	6.5-7 oz-eq.	7-7.5 oz-eq.	7-7.5 oz-eq.	7.5-8 oz-eq.
Milk	2-3 c.	3 c.	3 c.	3 c.	3 c.	3 c.	3 c.	3 c.
Healthy Oils	4 tsp.	5 tsp.	5 tsp.	6 tsp.	6 tsp.	7 tsp.	8 tsp.	8 tsp.

Day One

FOOD CHOICES

Breakfast: _____   Lunch: _____

Dinner: _____   Snacks: _____

Group	Fruits	Vegetables	Grains	Meat & Beans	Milk	Oils
Goal Amount						
Estimate Your Total						
Increase ⇧ or Decrease ⇩ ?						

PHYSICAL ACTIVITY

Description: _____

Steps/Miles/Minutes: _____

SPIRITUAL ACTIVITY

Description: _____

Day Two

FOOD CHOICES

Breakfast: _____   Lunch: _____

Dinner: _____   Snacks: _____

Group	Fruits	Vegetables	Grains	Meat & Beans	Milk	Oils
Goal Amount						
Estimate Your Total						
Increase ⇧ or Decrease ⇩ ?						

PHYSICAL ACTIVITY

Description: _____

Steps/Miles/Minutes: _____

SPIRITUAL ACTIVITY

Description: _____

Day Three

FOOD CHOICES

Breakfast: _____   Lunch: _____

Dinner: _____   Snacks: _____

Group	Fruits	Vegetables	Grains	Meat & Beans	Milk	Oils
Goal Amount						
Estimate Your Total						
Increase ⇧ or Decrease ⇩ ?						

PHYSICAL ACTIVITY

Description: _____

Steps/Miles/Minutes: _____

SPIRITUAL ACTIVITY

Description: _____

Day Four

FOOD CHOICES

Breakfast: _____ Lunch: _____

Dinner: _____ Snacks: _____

Group	Fruits	Vegetables	Grains	Meat & Beans	Milk	Oils
Goal Amount						
Estimate Your Total						
Increase ⇧ or Decrease ⇩ ?						

PHYSICAL ACTIVITY

Description: _____

Steps/Miles/Minutes: _____

SPIRITUAL ACTIVITY

Description: _____

_____

Day Five

FOOD CHOICES

Breakfast: _____ Lunch: _____

Dinner: _____ Snacks: _____

Group	Fruits	Vegetables	Grains	Meat & Beans	Milk	Oils
Goal Amount						
Estimate Your Total						
Increase ⇧ or Decrease ⇩ ?						

PHYSICAL ACTIVITY

Description: _____

Steps/Miles/Minutes: _____

SPIRITUAL ACTIVITY

Description: _____

_____

Day Six

FOOD CHOICES

Breakfast: _____ Lunch: _____

Dinner: _____ Snacks: _____

Group	Fruits	Vegetables	Grains	Meat & Beans	Milk	Oils
Goal Amount						
Estimate Your Total						
Increase ⇧ or Decrease ⇩ ?						

PHYSICAL ACTIVITY

Description: _____

Steps/Miles/Minutes: _____

SPIRITUAL ACTIVITY

Description: _____

_____

Day Seven

FOOD CHOICES

Breakfast: _____ Lunch: _____

Dinner: _____ Snacks: _____

Group	Fruits	Vegetables	Grains	Meat & Beans	Milk	Oils
Goal Amount						
Estimate Your Total						
Increase ⇧ or Decrease ⇩ ?						

PHYSICAL ACTIVITY

Description: _____

Steps/Miles/Minutes: _____

SPIRITUAL ACTIVITY

Description: _____

_____

Live It Tracker

Name: _____   My week at a glance: ☐ Great ☐ So-so ☐ Not so great

Date: _____ Week #: _____ Calorie Range: _____   My food goal for next week: _____

Activity Level: None, < 30 min/day, 30-60 min/day, 60+ min/day   My activity goal for next week: _____

Scripture Memory Verse: _____

RECOMMENDED DAILY AMOUNT OF FOOD FROM EACH GROUP

Group	Daily Calories							
	1300-1400	1500-1600	1700-1800	1900-2000	2100-2200	2300-2400	2500-2600	2700-2800
Fruits	1.5-2 c.	1.5-2 c.	1.5-2 c.	2-2.5 c.	2-2.5 c.	2.5-3.5 c.	3.5-4.5 c.	3.5-4.5 c.
Vegetables	1.5-2 c.	2-2.5 c.	2.5-3 c.	2.5-3 c.	3-3.5 c.	3.5-4.5 c.	4.5-5 c.	4.5-5 c.
Grains	5 oz-eq.	5-6 oz-eq.	6-7 oz-eq.	6-7 oz-eq.	7-8 oz-eq.	8-9 oz-eq.	9-10 oz-eq.	10-11 oz-eq.
Meat & Beans	4 oz-eq.	5 oz-eq.	5-5.5 oz-eq.	5.5-6.5 oz-eq.	6.5-7 oz-eq.	7-7.5 oz-eq.	7-7.5 oz-eq.	7.5-8 oz-eq.
Milk	2-3 c.	3 c.	3 c.	3 c.	3 c.	3 c.	3 c.	3 c.
Healthy Oils	4 tsp.	5 tsp.	5 tsp.	6 tsp.	6 tsp.	7 tsp.	8 tsp.	8 tsp.

Day One

FOOD CHOICES

Breakfast: _____   Lunch: _____

Dinner: _____   Snacks: _____

Group	Fruits	Vegetables	Grains	Meat & Beans	Milk	Oils
Goal Amount						
Estimate Your Total						
Increase ⇧ or Decrease ⇩ ?						

PHYSICAL ACTIVITY

Description: _____

Steps/Miles/Minutes: _____

SPIRITUAL ACTIVITY

Description: _____

Day Two

FOOD CHOICES

Breakfast: _____   Lunch: _____

Dinner: _____   Snacks: _____

Group	Fruits	Vegetables	Grains	Meat & Beans	Milk	Oils
Goal Amount						
Estimate Your Total						
Increase ⇧ or Decrease ⇩ ?						

PHYSICAL ACTIVITY

Description: _____

Steps/Miles/Minutes: _____

SPIRITUAL ACTIVITY

Description: _____

Day Three

FOOD CHOICES

Breakfast: _____   Lunch: _____

Dinner: _____   Snacks: _____

Group	Fruits	Vegetables	Grains	Meat & Beans	Milk	Oils
Goal Amount						
Estimate Your Total						
Increase ⇧ or Decrease ⇩ ?						

PHYSICAL ACTIVITY

Description: _____

Steps/Miles/Minutes: _____

SPIRITUAL ACTIVITY

Description: _____

Day Four

FOOD CHOICES

Breakfast: _____ Lunch: _____

Dinner: _____ Snacks: _____

Group	Fruits	Vegetables	Grains	Meat & Beans	Milk	Oils
Goal Amount						
Estimate Your Total						
Increase ⇧ or Decrease ⇩ ?						

PHYSICAL ACTIVITY

Description: _____

Steps/Miles/Minutes: _____

SPIRITUAL ACTIVITY

Description: _____

_____

Day Five

FOOD CHOICES

Breakfast: _____ Lunch: _____

Dinner: _____ Snacks: _____

Group	Fruits	Vegetables	Grains	Meat & Beans	Milk	Oils
Goal Amount						
Estimate Your Total						
Increase ⇧ or Decrease ⇩ ?						

PHYSICAL ACTIVITY

Description: _____

Steps/Miles/Minutes: _____

SPIRITUAL ACTIVITY

Description: _____

_____

Day Six

FOOD CHOICES

Breakfast: _____ Lunch: _____

Dinner: _____ Snacks: _____

Group	Fruits	Vegetables	Grains	Meat & Beans	Milk	Oils
Goal Amount						
Estimate Your Total						
Increase ⇧ or Decrease ⇩ ?						

PHYSICAL ACTIVITY

Description: _____

Steps/Miles/Minutes: _____

SPIRITUAL ACTIVITY

Description: _____

_____

Day Seven

FOOD CHOICES

Breakfast: _____ Lunch: _____

Dinner: _____ Snacks: _____

Group	Fruits	Vegetables	Grains	Meat & Beans	Milk	Oils
Goal Amount						
Estimate Your Total						
Increase ⇧ or Decrease ⇩ ?						

PHYSICAL ACTIVITY

Description: _____

Steps/Miles/Minutes: _____

SPIRITUAL ACTIVITY

Description: _____

_____

let's count our miles!

Join the 100-Mile Club this Session

Can't walk that mile yet? Don't be discouraged! There are exercises you can do to strengthen your body and burn those extra calories. Keep a record on your Live It Tracker of the number of minutes you do these common physical activities, convert those minutes to miles following the chart below, and then mark off each mile you have completed on the chart found on the back of the front cover. Report your miles to your 100-Mile Club representative when you first arrive each week. Remember, you are not competing with anyone else . . . just yourself. Your job is to strive to reach 100 miles before the last meeting in this session. You can do it—just keep on moving!

Walking

slowly, 2 mph	30 min. = 156 cal. = 1 mile
moderately, 3 mph	20 min. = 156 cal. = 1 mile
very briskly, 4 mph	15 min. = 156 cal. = 1 mile
speed walking	10 min. = 156 cal. = 1 mile
up stairs	13 min. = 159 cal. = 1 mile

Running/Jogging
10 min. = 156 cal. = 1 mile

Cycling Outdoors

slowly, <10 mph	20 min. = 156 cal. = 1 mile
light effort, 10-12 mph	12 min. = 156 cal. = 1 mile
moderate effort, 12-14 mph	10 min. = 156 cal. = 1 mile
vigorous effort, 14-16 mph	7.5 min. = 156 cal. = 1 mile
very fast, 16-19 mph	6.5 min. = 152 cal. = 1 mile

Sports Activities

Playing tennis (singles)	10 min. = 156 cal. = 1 mile
Swimming	
light to moderate effort	11 min. = 152 cal. = 1 mile
fast, vigorous effort	7.5 min. = 156 cal. = 1 mile
Softball	15 min. = 156 cal. = 1 mile
Golf	20 min. = 156 cal = 1 mile
Rollerblading	6.5 min. = 152 cal. = 1 mile
Ice skating	11 min. = 152 cal. = 1 mile

Jumping rope   7.5 min. = 156 cal. = 1 mile
Basketball   12 min. = 156 cal. = 1 mile
Soccer (casual)   15 min. = 159 cal. = 1 mile

Around the House
Mowing grass   22 min. = 156 cal. = 1 mile
Mopping, sweeping, vacuuming   19.5 min. = 155 cal. = 1 mile
Cooking   40 min. =160 cal. = 1 mile
Gardening   19 min. = 156 cal. = 1 mile
Housework (general)   35 min. = 156 cal. = 1 mile
Ironing   45 min. = 153 cal. = 1 mile
Raking leaves   25 min. = 150 cal. = 1 mile
Washing car   23 min. = 156 cal. = 1 mile
Washing dishes   45 min. = 153 cal. = 1 mile

At the Gym
Stair machine   8.5 min. = 155 cal. = 1 mile
Stationary bike
  slowly, 10 mph   30 min. = 156 cal. = 1 mile
  moderately, 10-13 mph   15 min. = 156 cal. = 1 mile
  vigorously, 13-16 mph   7.5 min. = 156 cal. = 1 mile
  briskly, 16-19 mph   6.5 min. = 156 cal. = 1 mile
Elliptical trainer   12 min. = 156 cal. = 1 mile
Weight machines (used vigorously)   13 min. = 152 cal.=1 mile
Aerobics
  low impact   15 min. = 156 cal. = 1 mile
  high impact   12 min. = 156 cal. = 1 mile
  water   20 min. = 156 cal. = 1 mile
Pilates   15 min. = 156 cal. = 1 mile
Raquetball (casual)   15 min. = 159 cal. = 1 mile
Stretching exercises   25 min. = 150 cal. = 1 mile
Weight lifting (also works for weight
  machines used moderately or gently)   30 min. = 156 cal. = 1 mile

Family Leisure
Playing piano   37 min. = 155 cal. = 1 mile
Jumping rope   10 min. = 152 cal. = 1 mile
Skating (moderate)   20 min. = 152 cal. = 1 mile
Swimming
  moderate   17 min. = 156 cal. = 1 mile
  vigorous   10 min. = 148 cal. = 1 mile
Table tennis   25 min. = 150 cal. = 1 mile
Walk/run/play with kids   25 min. = 150 cal. = 1 mile

Week 2: Not Beyond Our Reach

Now what I am commanding you today is not too difficult for you or beyond your reach.

Week 3: Words for the Wise Traveler

It is better not to vow than to make a vow and not fulfill it.

Daily Victory, Daily Joy

Daily Victory, Daily Joy
Scripture Memory Verses:

DEUTERONOMY 30:11
ECCLESIASTES 5:5
1 PETER 5:8
2 CORINTHIANS 10:4
JEREMIAH 33:3

2 CORINTHIANS 5:9
ACTS 20:24
ZECHARIAH 4:6
ROMANS 8:1
PSALM 9:10

How to Use These Cards:

Separate cards from the Bible study book. These cards are designed to be used when exercising. To do this, you may want to punch a hole in the upper left corner of the cards and place on a ring. When you have finished memorizing all the verses from one study, add the new Bible study cards to the ring and continue practicing the old verses while learning the new ones. Cards may be placed anywhere you will see them regularly—on the dashboard of your car, on a mirror, on a desk. After you have memorized the verse, begin using the reverse side of the card so the reference is connected to the verse. This is a great way to practice the verses you have already learned.

DEUTERONOMY 30:11

ECCLESIASTES 5:5

4 health
first place
discover a new way to healthy living

Week 6: Pave the Pathway with Prayer

Call to me and I will answer you and tell you great and unsearchable things you do not know.

Week 7: Living a Life Pleasing to God

We make it our goal to please him, whether we are at home in the body or away from it.

Week 4: Friends and Foes

Be self-controlled and alert. Your enemy the devil prowls around like a roaring lion looking for someone to devour.

Week 5: Our Battle Hymn

The weapons we fight with are not the weapons of the world. On the contrary, they have divine power to demolish strongholds.

JEREMIAH 33:3

1 PETER 5:8

2 CORINTHIANS 5:9

2 CORINTHIANS 10:4

Week 10: Jesus Paid It All

Therefore, there is now no condemnation for those who are in Christ Jesus.

Week 11: Trust in the Lord

Those who know your name will trust in you, for you, Lord, have never forsaken those who seek you.

Week 8: Completing the Task

However, I consider my life worth nothing to me, if only I may finish the race and complete the task the Lord Jesus has given me—the task of testifying to the gospel of God's grace.

Week 9: Our Power Supply

"Not by might nor by power, but by my Spirit," says the Lord Almighty.

ROMANS 8:1

ACTS 20:24

PSALM 9:10

ZECHARIAH 4:6